# Natural Healing
# with
# Herbal Combinations

Brian Wright

GREEN
LIBRARY

First Impression 1984
Revised and Updated Edition 1990
Copyright © Brian Wright 1984, 1990

Designed and illustrated by David Simpson
ISBN 0/946170/01/0

Green Library
Mariner's House
53a High Street
Bagshot, Surrey

Printed on recycled paper

# Contents

# Acknowledgements

Any writer in the field of herbs and healing must be aware of an immense history of human involvement through masterpieces of written work, inspired experimentation and the accumulation of human experience. So my first thanks must go to those herbalists, human scientists and healers who provide us with a wealth of observation and experience.

I must also give thanks for the contribution of friends and clients who have been courageous enough to use herbal and nutritional methods in a time when our conventional training is to mistrust such "unsanctioned" ways. However, I believe that the time of ascendancy of the current benighted view of the body, its science, needs and medicine is practically over, and look forward to the time when humanity can look after its health in a more harmonious and respectful way.

I cannot claim originality in any way for the contents of the book. The herbal combinations themselves are in a tradition of North American and European herbalism, and they were originally suggested by the herbalist and healer Marshall Lever. Information on the herbs comes from traditional herbals, some modern experimental evidence and my own and others' experience with them over more than ten years. The physiology comes from textbooks, but the intention here is to give an outline which ordinary people can comprehend and use in relation to their own health. The approach to natural healing is in line with naturopathy, nutrition and orthomolecular medicine, and modern herbalism. The underlying philosophy and the basis for my approach to health and life comes from my involvement with Arica and the enlightened teacher, Oscar Ichazo. I have no doubt that his experience of the transcendental, which led to the logic of cycles, Trialectics, and a real method for clarifying consciousness and achieving enlightenment, is changing our society profoundly.

For ten years of close working companionship I would like to give my appreciation to my wife Celia and to David Simpson.

The information presented in this book is purely educational. Any treatment is undertaken entirely on the reader's responsibility. If diagnosis or medical treatment is required, it should be performed by a practitioner, preferably one oriented to and knowledgeable in natural medicine

# Preface

Helping people to find their nature and explore their nature, With Nature, is a beautiful thing. This is what Brian Wright has done again in this new edition of "Natural Healing with Herbal Combinations".

To be able to trust that plants can heal is a precious gift. Brian's enthusiasm and generous way of relating, makes finding that trust easier; he shows a positive road, yet allows you to walk it for yourself.

There is nothing more delightful than to use what springs from the Earth to heal. Plants have a knack of not just penetrating every organ and system but our very souls as well. They are the truly wholistic healers, who invite us to share their joys and awareness.

This book will inspire and urge you to explore many possibilities for loving, nurturing and healing your body with Natures help.

**Jill Davies**
*Author and Herbalist*

# Enjoying Herbs and Health

What could be more beautiful and inspiring than to spend one's time surrounded by plants of great variety and vibrancy which happen, in this wondrous Creation, to heal people? What could be more worthwhile than to help ourselves and others be well?

With similar emotions and good intentions, many of us embark on learning about herbs and health. But isn't it difficult? The herbs don't yield up their secrets of themselves, it's often difficult to distinguish what is happening if you become your own guineapig, and the herbal books are mainly too full of detail or too sparse in information about the body.

Equally, if your interest is in natural healing and how the body works, the number of pieces in the jigsaw are too large. It includes theories of health, books on physiology and biochemistry, medicine and a good deal of training of the senses.

Having covered a lot of this area myself, I wanted to write a book about a small number of tried herbal combinations, and really try to give some insight into how they work and how to amplify their effects. Combinations offer the possibility of concentrating some of the effects of the herbs while having a wide spread of benefits. This book is a "nutritional healer's" approach rather than a herbalist's because there is more emphasis on the actual healing effects than in identifying new herbs and finding very specific cures. This approach also involves a fresh look at what our complex and miraculous human body is about.

It seems that the language for talking about natural healing is undergoing a great process of change and clarification. I think we are at the beginning of a shift of view in the body sciences as extraordinary as that which followed Einstein in the physical sciences. It's an exciting time! Just as physics has to work on the interface with metaphysics, so healing has to work with intuition and mystical perception of the body as well as with science. As I edit the second edition I am aware that the voices that would like to put health back into a Dark Age of superstition and fear (based on the assumption that allopathic medicine is the standard for

7

medicine and science and that everything else is quackery) are growing strident.

It has become absolutely evident in the last few years that the factors which are threatening the balance of Nature in the planet - climatic change, radiation from nuclear plant accidents and weapons testing, pollution of our land, water, air, and oceans, and the rapid damage to the ionosphere, forests etc. - are also affecting us. Humanity is threatened by overpopulation and famine, we all exist in conditions of stress, our immunity is easily compromised and new diseases are arising to which there is no allopathic answer.

In the midst of this crisis of survival the least we can do is to take care of our health in a natural harmonious way. Ordinary people are using herbal and other natural healing methods in quite sophisticated ways to improve their health and their whole ability to function and express their potential. The other message of this book is that you can do it too!

# Part One

## Herbs and Healing - Basic Questions

# What is the Body?

**Responsibility**

Everyone reading this book has begun to leave behind that childlike lack of responsibility for their own body. Whenever I hear "Doctor says I should have it out", or "They say there's nothing much wrong with me", or "I feel so much safer on antibiotics for my cold", it reminds me of times when I was told I might get polio if I didn't have an injection, and completely believed I would be stricken by it the following day. Whereas the belief that reality is dictated by parents goes quite quickly, the higher authority of "experts" lasts a long time, particularly when it comes to that mysterious thing, the human body.

We learn quite easily to accept responsibility for our possessions or our work. For instance, most of us drive a car without having a permanent instructor by our sides, and we turn up to work without having to be collected. But with our bodies we constantly forget that medical diagnosis and advice is a service for us, and we can use health experts exactly as we might engage a solicitor, architect or plumber for professional help.

Recognising that our bodies are the only things we can really say are ours, we must take responsibility for what happens to them. We can't have freedom of action without taking responsibility. To take responsibility we must know some basic laws of the body. Otherwise information about herbs and healing means as little as a book of computer maintenance would to someone born in the Middle Ages.

Our bodies are such wonders of creation that they can be an endless source of fascination, such vast containers that they can hold unlimited joy and love, and such good transmitters that they can allow complete expression of human creativity. The alternative to getting to know ourselves is to live with minimal feeling, as if anaesthetised, or to live in pain. Who would choose that way?

So before we look at the herbal healers, let's consider the organism they are meant to heal - the human body.

**Body Feeling**

Our bodies normally work so efficiently that we don't have to attend to them at all. In fact most people remain completely unaware that they are in this amazing biological

11

organism until they have a pain or another strong feeling.

Pain is normally regarded as a distressing phenomenon which needs to be suppressed immediately. But from the body's point of view it is a way of attracting our attention, pointing out that something is wrong, out of balance. In any natural healing method, the attitude of suppression is replaced by more careful listening to the body and an active interest in the meaning of feelings from it. If we can monitor the early stages of imbalance we can act quickly before pain or illness takes hold. Without becoming hypochodriacs we can use this increasing sensitivity to keep ourselves in a much better state of health and energy.

Everyone knows that in music, dance, visual art, a personal relationship or religious experience, as we get more in touch with our feelings, we become more sensitive and accurate. The body is an instrument which allows internal monitoring of its states. We have a great variety of internal nerve receptors for pressure, temperature, muscle stretch and relaxation and so on. Also it has been recognised in methods of development of awareness, such as yoga or the Taoist traditions [1], that the body can be trained to feel itself in complete detail. We cannot afford to ignore this training of perception through visualisation, because it is a matter of experience that the more awareness there is of the inside, the more complete our view of the outside world is. In other words developing our ability to feel our bodies from the inside will amplify our knowledge of health, herbs and all the processes of Nature.

So when next you get an odd or uncomfortable feeling, be sure that it is not indicating a deficiency of aspirin, but that it might be telling you something about the way you have been treating your body. It might be possible to improve the balance of your life and to use harmonious ways to deal with discomfort. The better we know our body, the more accurate we will be in rebalancing it.

## Body Science

The sciences of the human body are about to undergo a revolution. Not a violent one, because the seeds of change are long planted. And not one where the old knowledge is lost, because the revolution will really happen in underlying viewpoint rather than in the details of discovery.

The old way of science has been to analyse in finer and finer detail, so that the branches of the tree of knowledge have become more and more finely divided. This approach has made sciences like Anatomy, Physiology and Biochemistry a life's work to comprehend. The new science recognises that knowledge like a tree has cycles of growth, and fits into an ecological pattern. For instance it is quite possible to read a physiology textbook in which information about the role of vitamin C in the adrenal glands is completely disconnected from information about stress. This ignores the fact that vitamin C is one of the primary resources needed to make adrenal hormones, and that adrenal hormones are central in controlling a whole spectrum of stress reactions. Old science splits the understanding of concepts like "vitamin C", "adrenal glands" and "stress" into separate compartments.

The new science takes its starting point as the recognition that the body is a whole, existing in different levels - molecules, cells, organs, systems etc - which are interdependent. Just as minerals, flora and fauna make up the ecology of an area, so the levels of the body make up an ecologically whole organism.

This book is for people who have no specialised knowledge of body science. But if, like me, you have an active curiosity in this area it is a very good idea to have some basic maps to avoid confusion. Then all the work and intense effort of researchers can be built into a picture that means something to us in our own bodies and during the course of our own natural healing.

## The Practical Way

The only practical way to understand the body is to start with one's own experience and to work toward seeing the thread that runs through it, to gather the meaning of it.

Let's consider the mysterious subject of diagnosis. The fact that all doctors, whether of Western medicine, acupuncture or "primitive" magical medicine, spend a lot of time learning very complex and mysterious methods of diagnosis is off putting to most people. It is easy to forget that with nearly all illnesses or minor imbalances, the information from body feelings and objective symptoms points straight to a major body system.

In self-healing the first concern is to strengthen and rebalance the whole body. Secondly there is usually a focus which needs healing, for instance in the digestive system. Thirdly we might want to consider an organ, (the stomach perhaps), a tissue (the stomach lining), a molecular imbalance (loss of protein) or an energy imbalance (the effect of stress on the stomach) in more detail. Here we can use our detective's nose to examine the details, and bring in the information from past history, expert opinion and so on.

If the person has stomach ulcers, diagnosed and plainly seen in X-rays, that is very useful information. But other relevant facts are his stress level, the use of protein in other parts of the body, diet and the conditions under which he eats, condition of similar tissues (the skin and other 'linings'), his emotional state and his history. We can be sure that he developed stomach ulcers through imbalances in his life and we remain most interested in his digestive system as a whole and his nutrition. The intention of a natural healing method would be to rebalance all the factors involved so that the pattern producing ulcers is eliminated. At the same time we would hope to aid the healing of the ulcers themselves.

We should also not be foxed by the complicated names given to diseases. Diseases are neither entities in themselves, nor states we need to fight and destroy, they are the description of our body-out-of-balance. So the knowledge we need to understand disease is sympathetic self-knowledge, or empathy.

The key to practical action in natural healing is empathy. There was never a truer saying than "Physician, heal thyself", because empathy allows us to know from the inside, not only about ourselves, but about others.

We use empathy every day. For instance when driving, we have to realise that other drivers are like ourselves. They have the ability to judge distances, steer and control the car, pace themselves with other vehicles, respond to signals and signs. They have desires to drive fast, daringly or carefully, and to stay alive. If we did not have a good idea of what kind of beings were in the other driving seat, we would really be in trouble.

We can combine scientific analysis and our ability to compare one feeling or experience with another, and then the third type of reason, empathy, which allows us to act with confidence (2). This is easier to see if we look at healing a simpler organism, like a houseplant. Suppose its leaf tips are brown. If this is the limit of the damage, we can compare with previous experience. "This is the same as happened last year with Mrs Smith's plant". Then we may refer to a book and check the symptoms with an analysis of plant illnesses. We should then have a series of alternative explanations and remedies. This is the point at which we need to empathise, to see ourselves in the place of the plant. "The amount of water seems OK, the soil feels adequate, but there is a draught from the window". This fits with our other explanations, so we act with reasonable certainty in removing the plant from the draught. The same type of three-stage reasoning is basic to all complete healing whether healing oneself or others.

In this book you will find a basic scientific description of the body in relation to herbs. You will find comparisons, and analogies which might relate to feelings and past experiences. You will find recommendations for action, using herbs, nutrition, other therapies and exercise. All you need to supply is the capacity to empathise, to see yourself in the descriptions and stories, to see how the other parts of the picture apply to you, and to see yourself as capable of transforming your health.

## Basic Maps

Einstein maintained that all scientists begin with a belief or model (we might say, map), and that this preconceived view determines to a major extent what they actually find [3]. Numerous experiments in Psychology have shown that our expectations and beliefs are the most important factors in deciding on what is relevant in any investigation, and in determining how we set up an experiment and interpret the results. So we must conclude that if a whole view of healing and well-being is the required result, we must start with a map of the whole area. We must lay out pre- conceived ideas and try to avoid inaccuracies from the beginning.

The different areas of knowledge, like Biochemistry, Psychology, Philosophy and the Arts, can appear to be overwhelmingly chaotic in their diversity without a map. The body itself often appears to be a worse problem to comprehend. If we believe that Mind is separate from Body, for example, all kinds of healing and harmonising methods become impossible to use - we simply cannot see how they could work. For instance, I heard on the radio a doctor categorically denying that diet had any effect on depression. In the face of fairly straightforward evidence she simply could not accept that diet could have an effect since depression was not even in the same class of ideas as food. In other words her map of health did not include both "depression" and "food".

In biological sciences, Charles Darwin's vision of the

progress of evolution from simple forms to ever more complex forms of life, has been compelling [4]. It may have been that he was wrong about many of the details of the theory, and the view is in need of thorough revision [5], but his vision revolutionised Biology because it located all the species of animals and plants in one comprehensive map.

The map we use takes as its basis the idea that matter manifests at different levels. The body is made of energy condensed into matter. The most basic level of matter is that of the *subatomic particles* - that strange family of dots and squiggles studied by atom-smashing physicists. These get together in regular configurations, known as *atoms*. The body's atoms are of particular types - carbon, oxygen, nitrogen, hydrogen, calcium and so on, which combine together in *molecules*. Biochemistry is the study of the millions of interactions between molecules which allow us to build up specialised body structures and functions and a means of reproducing whole living systems. Some of the most important body molecules are composed of proteins, fats and carbohydrates, vitamins and minerals. They make up structures like cell walls and nuclei, and molecules like enzymes which determine all the biochemical functions of the body.

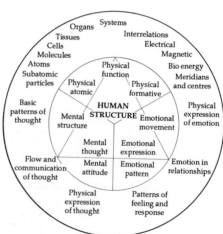

The unit which expresses the outcome of biochemical activity is the *cell*. Cells specialise and are organised into *tissues* to cover bodily functions like forming membranes (skins) or communications networks (nerve tissue). Tissues make up structures which have quite individual characteristics, like the liver, kidneys, heart and so on, and these *organs* accomplish major tasks for the body. *Systems* are the expression of a higher level of organisation still, giving the body the total capability of digestion, protection, movement, circulation, and so on. Science does not yet take us further, but we can complete our map from other sources while we expect scientists to follow more carefully with observation and experiments.

Systems interrelate and balance their functions according to the whole body's requirement of coping with a changing environment. There are *electrical* and *magnetic* relationships between systems, and then the level of *bio-energy* or chi-energy which is understood in Chinese culture through Acupuncture (6) as the level which describes the meeting point between the "gross physical body" and formative higher energies. At a higher level of organisation we come to the way the body is used in emotional life. In the centre of the emotional world we have the way emotion is expressed, and the way we feel it as impulse. The language we use points to the fact that emotion is still a level of manifesting matter/energy. We talk of heavy feelings and light heartedness.

When we look at our emotional life, we see patterns - ups and downs, feelings that come up again and again. Emotional patterns are immediately related to mental attitude, the level at which beliefs, attitudes and decisions control the emotional pattern. In the centre of the emotional realm comes thought and understanding, at the upper level comes the mental structure and patterns which underlie the way we think. This map itself can be seen at this level.

Beyond the mental realm we come to the spiritual realm. Although this book concentrates on the physical aspects of health, all four realms are related and for complete healing must be taken together.

At each level of manifestation there are regular happenings which can be explained by scientific or natural laws. Each is a subject for scientific investigation, artistic expression and self-awareness. Between the levels there is a hierachy of organisation. For instance cells are organised into tissue types, and organs are made up of tissues in specific formats.

Between elements there is correlation and the expression of harmony or disharmony. For instance water retention in all body cells may be correlated with a tendency to hold on to emotion, not express it physically, and with difficulty in decision making. So on the map we can see how some of the sciences and arts of the human being work lawfully on their own level and how there are connections between adjacent ones, like Biochemistry and Physiology. In addition to this kind of relationship a healing practice like Homeopathy ⁊ has a harmony of effects in bodily, emotional, mental and spiritual patterns, and treatment actually works through the patterning in each realm.

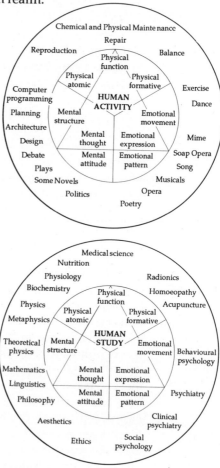

You are invited to take these maps as a starting point for thinking about what the relationships between structures, activities and studies are The maps are designed to make it easier to think of the whole sphere of human structure and activity and stimulate a truly holistic view of health.

## Consciousness

What happens when we imagine removing all those layers of manifestation? This question has been asked throughout human history, and it is answered in mystical schools and genuine religious traditions. The Tibetan Book of the Dead [8] is one document giving advice on the dissolution of the layers of manifestation and how to maintain consciousness throughout. For whether this journey is undertaken during life or after death, consciousness is the ultimate, undefinable, remaining factor.

Consciousness is the axis of our map. When consciousness attracts to it a human body, it 'clothes itself' in spirit, mind, emotions and physical body. When consciousness reaches the most basic level of matter, we are conceived and born and we can start the journey of life. One goal of the journey, as I understand it, is to restore an awakened consciousness to all levels of our human manifestation.

Our main problem is how to awaken, stay conscious, and to stop ourselves "falling asleep" in the midst of life.

In the course of the journey we remember experiences that have brought disharmony and imbalance. Often, touching on the pain of such areas is enough to send us back to sleep, to those levels of consciousness where we live in illusion, veiled from the real world. How clearly can you remember the first time you felt hurt by someone you loved, for instance? Most of us spend much of our lives in the illusions of superstitious beliefs and fears, absolute dependence on the rules of society, beliefs in the ego, in ungrounded theories, disillusionment with the ego or in fighting ourselves [9]. The natural and full experience of life has been veiled because we are afraid it might be painful.

Getting ill can sometimes confront us with the fact that we allow illusory beliefs, fears and habits to control our lives. We naturally withdraw from our usual activities, pay more attention to our bodies, and try to simplify our lives. Besides encouraging us to wake up to the disharmonies in our lives, consciousness of the process of illness is the major factor allowing a natural recovery. For instance, by tracing back events where I felt failure and a lack of support in my life I helped myself recover from persistent backache.

## Correlations

My friend came toward me one day looking slow and depressed. She said, "I feel so slow and out of rhythm today. My thoughts are all jammed together. I can't get rid of all the rubbish my boss keeps feeding me".

Her language contained all the clues needed to suspect constipation. I took her for a large salad and gave her some Herbal D. As her digestive system cleared, so did her thoughts and feelings.

The words we use unconsciously are accurate indications of the correlations that exist between different realms. Think of all the times we can't "stomach" something, when we are "heartbroken" or we admire someone for their "guts". It is guaranteed that someone with arthritic stiffness has some corresponding lack of flexibility in their thoughts and feelings.

Knowledge of corresponding thoughts, feelings and bodily patterns is one of the most powerful tools for diagnosis. Once we are aware that there is no absolute separation between body, emotions mind and spirit, we can notice and use this correlation in our own healing.

# What is Health?

**Balance**

Having identified the unity and wholeness of the human body, we move to the principle of balance. If we want to make a seesaw, we have to balance the two halves of a plank on a pivot. The body is a living pivot for many essential balances.

We have to maintain our whole balance in so many ways from walking on our "back legs" to balancing weight loss with weight gain. A cell membrane controls the balance between useful cell substances on one side and secretions and eliminations on the other. The pressure must be equalised and the cell achieves this by pumping out excess sodium ions. Cells can actively pull in useful molecules and eliminate others, and a balance between assimilation and elimination must be maintained.

We have many agents of balance in the body - substances which make a "pivot" between two halves of a process. At a molecular level we would look at enzymes as the agents of balance; at a tissue level we might be more interested in hormones. In science this kind of balancing is called "homeostasis", maintaining a constant state. At the level of body systems, the feedback mechanisms and controls are quite sophisticated. For instance, blood sugar level is maintained within a limited range by pancreas hormones in conjunction with the secretions and activities of adrenals, liver, pituitary and hypothalamus.

The idea of sugar takes us to another realm, the emotional one. Sugar is one of the substances we use to compensate, to back away from the areas of emotional pain. We may be in pain because of mental patterns that were laid down in a moment of fear or panic. But only when we are ready can we look at the origin of the bad feeling. To maintain temporary balance we may have to compensate.

Sometimes sugar is a lot better than getting neurotic, taking it out on somebody else, or breaking out in psychosomatic symtoms [10].

For complete health we should be aware of all our balances. For instance, we exercise our personalities in various unbalanced ways; workaholics and cynics are suppressing the lazy and gullible sides of their nature; the tough exterior always hides a soft interior, and the sentimentalist is basically as hard as steel. So as we go about all the different sides of life, we are either balancing ourselves, or we are accumulating habits of mind and body, leading to imbalances that often underlie illness.

## Harmony

Nature is always in harmony. Other species live their lives, die their deaths, and make their contribution to the universe without argument. It is only human beings who can muddle and mismanage enough to live out of harmony.

Harmony is the *balance and interrelationship* of all the levels of the body. This internal harmony means that there is also harmony with other people and with the environment. Although in the course of life we can make harmony and dissonance as complex as musical symphonies, the body always knows the route back. The pattern of harmony is inbuilt. This is the basis upon which all natural medicine depends.

In conventional medicine the inbuilt wisdom of the body is constantly under-estimated. What medical science calls the "placebo effect", where we are tricked into believing that a neutral pill will cure us, and it does, is really an example of harmony being re-established between the mental and physical levels. "Spontaneous remission", far from being an accident or a kind of 'trick' by the patient on the doctor, is a reminder that the body does know its way back to harmony.

It does not have to be pushed, adjusted, guided or bullied.

Certain healing agents have a natural harmony with the body, and herbs are among those that reinforce the natural return to health.

## Health

Achieving a full and reasonable definition of health went out of fashion when, during the industrial revolution, medicine left the fold of natural philosophy and came under the spell of technical expedience. This allowed such extraordinary mistakes as the treatment of syphilis by mercury and a loss of faith in herbal remedies.

Natural medicine has never really achieved a full definition either, so we are left in a position of not knowing quite what is meant by health.

We could say that health is the state when the body as a whole, and in all its aspects works in harmony. But that does not account for change. The universe changes, the earth changes with weathering and cataclysm, society and its culture and politics changes much faster, and we personally change moment by moment. So health, too, must be a dynamic state which allows adaptation to new situations.

However, change is not random or accidental. Everything in the universe changes in pre-established, relatively predictable ways (11). If this were not true, science could not work. Imagine heating a kettle of water and finding we produced steam the first day, ice the second and little green bugs on the third! Although we do not have all the laws and descriptions of change, we know that in this, our only universe, there is an invariable pattern to all changes.

Health is often regarded as the opposite of disease. With this in mind, conventional medicine goes all out to attack and conquer disease. But opposites like this only exist in the mind. Is day opposed to night? Is life in contradiction to death? What is considered the "thesis and antithesis" is actually a cycle in which one state has the potential to change to another, and this cycle of change is an inbuilt part of the way reality works. For instance, try balancing a pencil on your finger. You will find that balance is succeeded by imbalance, you adjust your finger every time you feel the pencil going out of balance and the cycle returns to balance. So within health there is the potential of disease, and within disease the potential of health.

So far, then, we can see health as a cyclical state which

indicates our adaptability. But we do not simply circulate between health and illness, we also tend either to improve our overall functioning or go downhill. When we use foods, exercise, herbs and natural healing agents to support body harmony, health spirals upwards.

When we only use inputs like medical drugs that attack disease we are not supporting the underlying vitality and functioning of the body and the spiral of overall health can spin down. This brings in the concept of "evolution" as the recognition that we can have positivity and progress in cycles, just as there is evolution in plants and animals.

As humans we are a product of our society and its history, a product of culture. We could not live humanly without it. We absorb whatever is available and express our individuality through its language, customs, arts, sciences and technology. The evolution of our culture has reached a critical point. It seems that we have to choose between a downward path in which the lowest point is complete destruction of the world, and an upward path, the ultimate point of which would be the realisation that we are one humanity, one spirit. As more and more people look for personal fulfilment in their lives, it becomes more and more obvious that the destinies of individuals and of the whole human society are completely interlinked. Practically speaking, we cannot hope to be healthy if we are born and brought up breathing air polluted by a hundred factory chimneys. Nor can we deal with the problem of pollution unless we are clear about what is healthy and whether we want to go towards death or life.

Health is an aspect of fulfillment which must be in harmony with the positive evolution of the human race. Health is the kind of harmony within and between the body's patterns that allows us to take the next step, allows us to function fully in an evolving world.

Becoming healthier is a natural, lawful process of change. The negativity, infections and imbalances we experience in our lives give us the material to work on in the process of natural healing and gaining real self-knowledge. When that damage is healed, the experience enriches our understanding. For example, healing weak and 'furred-up' arteries gives an enormous appreciation of the energy, nourishment and good humour coming from a good blood supply.

**Transcendent Health**

There is a condition of the human body which is beyond ordinary health and disease. It exists when the body is so closely balanced, harmonised and synchronised with the universe that it becomes a perfect channel for higher energies. This is a completely *natural* state, and, in a sense this is what we have been created for. Not only saints can experience it. We have all experienced it fleetingly at some time, though we may not have been awake, or remember it. It is often seen in young children, pregnant mothers and those who have devoted their lives to something beyond the concerns of the ego, such as the wellbeing of humanity. As we become absorbed by the process of natural healing, we have more and more opportunity to experience it.

Allow yourself the possiblility, "I can have transcendent health".

# What is Illness?

When the route back to health and harmony is blocked or disrupted, there is a condition of disease. The body will use a variety of methods to overcome, adapt to, or avoid this area of imbalance. When these methods attract our attention we recognise ourselves as being ill.

It is most important to differentiate between the underlying disease condition, which we may have to learn to be aware of, and our body's reaction to the imbalance which may provoke the symptoms we normally complain of. For instance, shortness of breath, as a complaint, may not primarily be to do with the lungs, but may be due to hardening and narrowing of arteries affecting blood supply and the heart. We try to adapt to reduced blood by increasing oxygen supply, but the amount needed exceeds the ability to breathe it, and we feel short of breath. Let's avoid this confusion by concentrating first on the disease, and the underlying imbalance and then on the body's attempt to adapt, which produces symptoms.

Asking "what is the cause of this disease" is a little like asking for the cause of the current economic condition. Secondly it is impossible to find a single cause. The medical 'whodunnit', where a virus, or sometimes just an incomprehensible name is revealed as the culprit, has become part of the great mystification of medicine. Disease is a pattern of weaknesses in the whole physical-emotional-mental-spiritual body, and only when this weakness exists do we attract recognisable reactions and illness.

Most of us have the germs of the common cold inside us continuously in an inactive state. Supposing we are feeling depressed about work, and we compensate by eating lots of chocolate and neglecting our need for exercise and good food. Normally we cope with such nutritional imbalances by using our liver to neutralise and kidneys or colon to eliminate poisonous waste, but when we allow the germs to feed on our waste products, in our nose and throat, they begin to breed. Even then we have a backup system of white protective cells and an immune response to bring them under control, but if this goes on being overstretched we develop cold symtoms.

Let's look at the main factors behind the imbalances of disease.

## Toxicity

One agent of imbalance is toxicity, poison. Suppose we are given antibiotics as a young child. This may kill off invading bacteria, but it also kills essential intestinal bacteria, producing more toxicity and directly inhibits the formation of body protein, interrupting growth and repair and showing up in dull skin, hair and eyes. Our young liver may neutralise some antibiotic and it may be expelled through the kidneys. But in the need to cope with further challenges, the body may shunt off some into the fat tissues. Toxins tend to collect in the most unused and asleep areas of the body, where we are unconscious of their effects. Since poisons put us under stress we avoid releasing them into the blood stream and they may stay in the tissues for years.

Sometimes toxins will emerge through the skin in sweat or through spots and rashes. Sometimes they are released during colds, pneumonia and in other mucus borne ways. Sometimes they accumulate in organs (like tonsils) inhibiting them, or even incapacitating them so much that we are advised to have them removed. Sometimes they form the focus for vague symptoms which medicine has not recognised as a named disease, and sometimes they produce degenerative, even fatal, long term diseases. It seems likely that lead is an important factor in multiple sclerosis for example (12). Western diseases preceding death are now predominantly degenerative.

Physical toxins correspond with poisons in other realms.

25

It is not for nothing that we call thoughts and feelings "poisonous". Just as physical toxins hide in the body, so these other poisons hide in the subconscious. In the course of healing we may have to uncover them with courage and the clear light of consciousness.

## Sources of Toxicity

Toxicity comes to us through planet-wide pollution. DDT is found even in polar ice, and moves through the bodies of herbivores and carnivores. It has a very long life, which means that we can be receiving the results of crops being sprayed many years before. It causes liver damage, infertility and a host of other effects. Lead and gases in the air cause major health problems, not only to our city children but to everyone. Weedkillers and nitrate fertilisers in the earth, chemical waste in the sea and acid rain, and the growing level and threat of radioactivity, are all direct poisons which every human being now has to face.

Toxicity comes to us now in our food. With hardly a word of protest, our food has been adulterated with additives and preservatives to the extent that the average consumption of preservatives is upward of five pounds a year![13] Since many of these substances have only been in use for under 50 years, we have no idea what the long term effects could be. Some commonly used colouring agents are known carcinogens (cancer agents), and at the very least, preservatives tend to 'preserve' and immobilise the natural biochemistry of the body. Our water is contaminated with aluminium, causing flatulence, pancreas damage and in sufficient quantities, brain damage and senility.

Of course, we do not have to succumb to this toxicity. Our food should supply us with beneficial vitamins and minerals to counteract toxins, like vitamin C and calcium which help us to deal with lead. But as some oranges are now regularly found to contain hardly one molecule of vitamin C, perhaps we should not rely too heavily on a good diet.

Lack of vitamins and minerals, and over use of sugar and salt and other nutritionally void foods, are the sources of internal biochemical disruption which forces our body to produce its own toxic residues from food. Long term lack of essential nutrients will prevent the body making the full range of enzymes which means that processes like digestion will be incomplete. Food residues can provoke allergic reactions, block and take over whole areas of the body, or attract bacteria and viruses. The infectious diseases associated with these germs are our reactions to the extra toxins which they produce. You can see that blaming the latest virus is a lazy way to comprehend the process of disease!

## Stress and Tension

When we perceive an event as traumatic, damaging, we respond to this agent of imbalance by a series of reactions including tension, inflammation and glandular output (14). Physical shocks and traumas may be held in tensions and internal toxicity for a lifetime, making the whole body try to adapt around them. Just as you might double up with pain, so the muscles can compress and harden round the site of injury eventually numbing the area. Other kinds of injury are held in similar ways by the body. It is well known in the body therapy, *CHUA KA* (15) which works on the tension and toxins held in connective tissue, that emotional, mental and spiritual negativity is released throughout the 'undoing' of physical tensions.

If there is a local site of injury, the body responds by increasing the blood flow, the amount of connective tissue and protective white cells. If the intruding agent cannot be removed, it is likely to be cut off from the rest of the body by a cyst wall. This process is under the control of the hormones, particularly of the adrenal glands. Stress of all kinds is analogous to this penetration of the body's defences. We can allow thoughts and feelings to 'get to us' and provoke a stress reaction from the glandular system. This reaction is usually enough to change the situation and reduce the threat, but we tend more and more to live with a continuous level of stress which underlies many of the imbalances and diseases to which we are subject.

The consequence of constant stress is exhaustion of glands and nerves, and great imbalances in the blood contents which affect the whole body. Our ability to respond to infection is reduced, and we may start developing degenerative diseases. For instance, the adrenal glands may become exhausted through overuse in stress, a lack of nutrients, and overstimulation with salt and sugar. At the same time the blood has been carrying excess fats, cholesterol and minerals which accumulate in inflamed areas. Disrupted hormones allow inflammation in the joints, and they begin to seize up in the all-too familiar pattern of arthritis.

## MalNutrition

The body is built out of protein, fats, water and many more complex molecules which all have to come ultimately from food. Also the energy we need to sustain all our life processes comes from combining the sugars we derive from food with oxygen. Every stage of the complex process of making energetic human bodies out of food is controlled by a catalyst, or enzyme. In a sense it is enzymes and their blueprint in the genes that make us precisely as we are. Almost every enzyme is vitally linked with one or more minerals and/or vitamins, which by definition are substances we have to get from food intake.

Lack of any vital nutrient, or imbalance in the assimilation of nutrients, will inevitably lead to poor functioning and often contribute to disease.

## Ageing, Self-Destruction and Internal Balance

Attempting to prove that there was an inbuilt limit to a cell's life, Leonard Hayflick observed that all cell cultures died after the same limited number of divisions. When vitamin E was added to the nutrient mixture, however, the cells went on dividing healthily far beyond the limits of experimental time [16]. It seems that any ideas of the inevitability of ageing must await the time when we have seen all the agents of imbalance removed.

A body free of toxicity, tension and stress and receiving optimum nutrition might go on until all the purposes in the emotional, mental and spiritual realms have been achieved. But here it is clear that the external sources of imbalance are not the only ones. The pattern of the metabolism, or energy circulation, in all the realms is immensely important.

Systems of healing like acupuncture address themselves directly to adjusting this internal flow of energy, with the knowledge that the body's response to external agents of imbalance will be improved correspondingly.

In the herbalists' tradition, some herbs are said to be 'emollient' (softening, promoting warmth and water), some 'refrigerant' (cooling) and others 'stimulant'. This system of thought conceives the body as consisting of energy with certain characteristics which require adjusting and balancing. The characteristics could be the '4 humours' which come down through Medieval medicine or the '5 elements' which come through Chinese medicine. Using herbs in this tradition requires a very particular training. Perhaps more useful to our current view of health is the idea that the body is continually adapting, and herbs are powerful aids to adaptation.

**Adaptation**     One of the overriding principles of the body is that whatever imbalance presents itself, there is an attempt to adapt. If a toxin disrupts a biochemical process, we try to neutralise or engulf the poison or bypass the process. If bacteria enter the body an inflammatory response takes blood, oxygen, white cells and mending protein to the area. If a gland becomes exhausted the rest of the system tries to compensate, for instance a low thyroid gland often provokes overactive adrenal glands - in other words we try to overcome the feeling of sluggishness with bursts of frenetic energy. If one of the B vitamins essential to energy production is in low supply, there is a build up of half-burnt sugars. We cope by storing this material or finding another way of breaking it down so that the missing link can be bypassed. Our bodies try to cope and maintain life to the last possible moment.

The adaptation is frequently taken for the illness. High temperature is a way of controlling the spread of infections since many viruses and bacteria are less active at a couple of degrees higher than normal, yet is regularly treated as a negative symptom in conventional medicine. It is obviously most important to look at the underlying agents of imbalance in treating disease, though we must understand how to support adaptive responses.

The scope of our adaptive responses is inbuilt. Whether we feel ill or not whilst adapting, depends a lot on the understanding we have of the process, and the support we give our bodies in terms of medicine, food, exercise and the whole pattern of life.

# How is Natural Health Restored?

In its most simple form, natural healing involves eliminating toxins, managing stress, improving nutrition and supporting adaptation. By the greatest good fortune, herbs help us in all these ways, and their effects are concentrated on the regions of the body most in need.

If we have the symptoms of catarrh, flu and 'runny' hayfever each year, toxicity is bound to be involved. It may originate in inadequate digestion, producing a build-up of hardened intestinal mucus. Incompletely digested foods and putrefaction enter the bloodstream and are taken to the liver. The liver is eventually overwhelmed and the mucus-laden toxins circulate in the blood and lymph reaching the whole body. The kidneys attempt to eliminate some of the poisons, and some is lost through sweat glands, but there is a build-up. These particular toxins are irritating, and produce inflammation in the sensitive membranes in the nose and lungs. So the natural treatment includes a cleansing starting from the digestive system, through blood and lymph, through liver, kidneys and skin, and especially through the nose, throat and lungs. Herbs are expert cleansers.

In this example, the stress response comes into the picture as the body's reaction to foreign particles in inflammatory hayfever. Building up the adrenal glands and pituitary, as well as the autonomic nerves would aid healing by controlling inflammation. Also we might expect infection to be better controlled, not only by reducing toxicity, but also by strengthening the thymus gland, centre of the immune system. This again depends on a reduction in overall stress. Herbs can be used to restore rhythm and strength to the glands and nerves.

Nutrition has to be considered in improving the state of digestion, but also in supplying the right nutrients to support healing and detoxification. Herbs can help here too by helping the body absorb and use vitamins and minerals.

The body's attempts to adapt have included the liver, kidneys, blood, lymph, skin, mucus membranes and glands. The functioning of each organ needs support, repair, stimulation, or harmonisation with feelings and thoughts. Herbs are perhaps the most direct natural way of dealing with specific organs or tissues. Because of their vibrational harmony with parts of the body, they can act as catalysts for positive change, and they can help the body as a whole to harmonise and adjust to these changes.

If we can interpret illness and symptoms as the outcome of disruption to the natural body processes, it is easy to see how every condition can be restored. Then we can really understand how to use herbs and other natural healers.

## Medicine

It has only been in the last century that the mania for medical scientific analysis in isolation has blinded us to maintaining health. Science, it has been said, is the knowledge of the one-eyed colourblind man. Certainly medical science has been obsessed by single causes, single disease entities, and single cures. 'Hard evidence' is asked of us complex human persons as if we were part of a game of celestial billiards, and our reactions were like the collisions between simple billiard balls.

In medicine the limited scientific view has led to more and more precise, but limited definitions of disease. Each disease has its special name, its virus, its own drug or surgical technique. The disease is seen as a thing to be fought and conquered. In cases of epidemics, wars and injury this view has produced spectacular cures and lifesaving drugs. The contribution of medicine to these areas is a great gift to us all. But somehow the patients never seem to be well! Drugs have toxic and highly stressful effects on the rest of the body. Surgery mends the particular, but maims the person as a whole.

It is this limitation in view which makes it important to reestablish the alternative to the current medical model. There are excellent doctors and medical scientists, but the established conventions and methods of training are dangerously out of balance. Doctors are trained only in disease, not in health; only in what food will keep people alive, not in nutrition for health; only in drugs and surgery, not in herbs and natural treatments.

## Drugs and Herbs

Powerful drugs can be extracted from herbs. Such drugs are good at healing certain symptoms, but often create more problems in the long term. Within their original herbs, drug molecules are much less disruptive. One example of this is the well known aspirin, used for decades to treat every ache, pain and cold symptom. Unfortunately it has destructive effects on the stomach lining which can lead to severe disruption of the digestive system and subsequently all the systems of the body. Yet the Greeks were using its source herb, the willow, for pain treatment 2400 years ago, and various species of the tree have been in use for centuries by North American Indians and Eurasian people, without noticeable side-effects [17].

One reason for the greater safety of herbs is that the concentration of the drug-like substance is far less. But, perhaps more importantly, the active substance is in a living relationship with other plant substances. The action of the whole is different from that of the sum of the parts. Another example of this difference occurs in homoeopathic medicine, where the active ingredient is dissolved in a regular and conscious way so many times that it is sometimes doubtful whether there is one molecule remaining in the final preparation. The effect of patterning the active agent in the whole mixture by the dissolving process seems to be the important aspect; a concept which is entirely foreign to our usual scientific understanding.

In the herbal combinations in this book there are none of the side effects we experience with medical drugs. As with all food substances some people may be allergic or sensitive to a herb, and others may not feel benefit, but usually there is simply a strengthening of the natural healing process.

## Food and Herbs

There is no reason to make an absolute distinction between food and herbs. We are born with a natural instinct to eat a diet which provides the right balance of biochemicals for our needs. That instinct usually gets distorted very quickly. Our senses and the delicate balance of energy are overwhelmed by being fed sugar, salt and a whole host of artificial preservatives, hormones and other chemicals. These set up patterns and habits of eating which over the long term make us ill. Food can certainly make us ill, and it can also make us better and help us maintain a good state of health. Hippocrates, famous for the oath which every doctor takes, was clear that diseases and cures came out of the natural conditions of life and said, 'Let food be your medicine and medicine be your food'.

Natural foods from plants contain the proteins, oils, starches and sugars needed for energy, building body cells, and for the millions of biochemical processes in the body. They also contain essential vitamins, minerals and other micronutrients with which the body manages all these processes. In addition plants have many substances which work in harmony with human biochemistry and which can modify some of these processes. When the modification causes problems we call these substances poisons. When it is helpful and harmonious we recognise healing properties. Many 'ordinary' foods have healing properties - onions, carrots, peppers, and so on. We can regard the herbal combinations as widening the range of beneficial foods we can have in our diet.

## Are Herbs Poisonous?

A one-sided approach to herbs will inevitably come to the wrong conclusions. Some government health departments have tried to ban the sale of comfrey on the grounds that the solanine it contains caused cancer when fed to rats. The amount fed to the rats was enormous, and as the originator of the Ames Test [18] for carcinogenicity discovered, many of our ordinary foods are carcinogenic when used above normal quantities. Coffee, mushrooms, parsnips, figs, cocoa, chocolate, alcohol, all food containing nitrite preservative (most meat), and all food containing nitrate fertiliser (most food except organically grown) have all been found to cause or exacerbate cancers. We do not develop cancers when eating better foods because they also have 'anticarcinogens' which are positively beneficial, according to Ames. The evidence of centuries of safe and effective comfrey use was simply ignored.

Another much publicised account of herb toxicity was originated in the report of a single case. The fact that such flagrantly unscientific work is taken seriously by doctors and scientific journals leads to the conclusion that science is not really the criterion when attacking 'alternative medicine'. The report was of 'mistletoe hepatitis' after mistletoe extract was taken for a few days [19]. The report did not state what other factors - drugs, pollutants, etc. - the woman in question had been exposed to or even what the other ingredients of the tablets were. In fact it has since been suggested that the tablets had no mistletoe in them at all. There are minute amounts of poisonous substances in mistletoe as in other herbs, but in such small quantities that correct dosage has produced no sign of toxicity in centuries of use.

A balanced attitude must recognise that herbs change the body's metabolism. When used as part of a healing and maintenance programme, these changes can be positive and helpful. When abused, even beneficial herbs can become dangerous if the quantities are large enough.

## Evidence that Herbs Heal

From the dawn of history mankind has recognised and remembered that certain plants are healing.

In the last few centuries, and particularly in the last one, recording and analysing has taken precedence over the direct recognition of that healing quality. Indeed, scientists, rationalists and doctors have generally done a good job of outlawing the idea that healing qualities can be recognised or perceived at all. Those who developed the skill of matching the plant to the person have been labelled sorcerers and witches or quacks and systematically destroyed, particularly in the West.

Now, I hope, we are entering an age when it is understood that the two views of herbs are not contradictory, but are both needed. In other words, knowledge is increased both through science and through developing perception. So to answer the question of finding evidence that herbs heal, besides our own experience we can look to two long traditions.

One is the careful recording of plants and their effects taken from other cultures and a tradition of clinical practice, represented by the great herbal encyclopaedias, like Mrs Grieve's Modern Herbal [20], which draws on several centuries' experience. In different times and places herbalists used different theories to help make the connection between the herb and the result of using it. For instance the classical Western set of elements - earth, water, air and fire - was written of by Aristotle. Galen, the prominent Medieval physician, combined the elements with the four humours, blood, phlegm, yellow bile and black bile, which were used by Hippocrates to describe types of balance in the body. Galenic doctors prescribed 'dry' remedies for 'moist' diseases, cold for hot and so on. Paracelsus overthrew this simplistic framework with his absolute commitment to actual results, real healing, and with his vast perception of mineral and chemical activity, psychology, astrology and alchemy [21]. Other herbalists, like Culpepper worked very successfully with clear observation and a theoretical basis of astrology. Herbalism in China has been highly successful for centuries and is based on similar ideas of elements and qualities. Since the nineteenth century there has been much more emphasis on anatomy and physiology, and the scientific approach to the effects of the chemical constituents of herbs. This evidence is increasingly backed by scientific experiments. Modern herbalists are well aware of the current scientific literature, which is growing despite the disparity in funding between herbal and pharmaceutical science.

The other tradition is that of the remarkable healers who refined their senses to a point where they could recognise the correct plant at the right time of day for a particular person with a unique set of imbalances. A wonderful recent example, is that of Edward Bach, a physician who, after a very success-ful career in conventional medicine, learned to recognise the healing qualities of flowers by touching them with his tongue and produced a set of remedies which work through the emotional pattern to undo disease states [22].

A complete herbalist has to combine these two ways with the third, self knowledge coming from personal experience.

## How do Herbs aid Healing?

There is no doubt that herbs aid the process of natural healing, and I have described four major components, detoxification, stress management, nutrition and strengthening adaptation. But there is a link missing in our understanding of how a plant and a body can be related so intimately. The drug-like effect of certain plant chemicals directly modifying metabolism is a part of that link, and the 'homoeopathic effect' (the patterning of active agents within a whole) can help us understand what is happening, but there is a possible third connection worth opening the mind to.

Science has taught us that all material things, including bodies and plants are made basically of the same material, certain subatomic particles. Perhaps the most basic particle is the photon, the 'packet' of light. But we find in some situations that light can only be interpreted as a wave formation, and we find that our 'objective' science is really built on the paradox that light is both particle and wave [23]. It is easy to imagine that the basic particles build up to produce atoms, molecules, bodies, plants and plantes. But what happens to the information held in the wave-form during this process?

In all mystical traditions, the human body is described in terms of light, colours. It is amply attested that perception can be developed to see colours beyond the normal range of vision [24]. Indeed there is an ancient tradition of teaching diagnosis by this means in Acupuncture Theory [25]. The harmony of wave-form, vibration or colour is the third major link between herbs and the human body, and it is this quality that can be perceived or intuited.

Lady's slipper has a vibrational connection with nerves, recognised in one of its names 'nerve-root'. There is often something else about the plant which suggests each use. For instance eyebright flowers are like little bright eyes and the herb is also vibrationally connected with the eyes. The so-called 'doctrine of signatures' was an attempt by herbalists to systematise similarities in structure between herbs and their target organs. It failed because the similarities are not in structure, but in vibration. The ability to see or intuit this kind of 'signature' needs to be trained.

**Visualisation and Intuition**

If you want to heal an organ or improve its functioning, it is known that a potent aid is to visualise the organ in perfect health. This is a good way to start gaining direct experience of the body which is needed to develop intuition in the area of herbs.

To begin, look at the most naturalistic drawing of the organ available. Locate it in your body. Spend two minutes, twice a day imagining that you can see the organ in its place in your body. Gradually fill in more detail. If it is the liver, for example, get to know how the lobes are arranged, the blood supply and the microscopic view so that you get a feeling for the type of cells. Find out what are its functions and what are its needs.

Soon you will begin to notice some feelings coming from the area, and it may remind you of experiences you have given it, you may give up some toxins, or improve its functioning. The idea is to begin to relate to your liver as a 'friend', rather than a mechanical object. Then you will know more directly what it needs, how it feels and 'thinks'. You may begin to get an idea of its colour, or at least have a feeling of its quality. Then you will be ready to listen to what your liver says about herbs! Just to be aware of an aspect of your body like this has an effect on health, as anyone with an experience of meditation can confirm.

The old herbalists really understood their herbs by watching them grow, seeing, smelling, tasting and touching them. As they cut, dried and prepared them, their senses would be completely open to them. This way of training the senses, without imposing ideas and beliefs on them, is the external complement to the internal visualisation which allows intuition to develop. Practice in seeing, hearing, smelling, tasting and using all the senses, without getting caught up in naming and categorising, will help build the openness needed to develop intuition.

**What is the Process of Getting Well?**

Being healthy is not just a matter of not feeling ill. It involves the whole body working well, harmoniously and with full energy. We can feel this kind of fulfilment and capacity for enjoyment!

Talking about getting well is always far more complicated than actually doing it, and it is often much more important to simply have the feeling of getting more healthy rather than understanding the minute processes involved. If every time you have a symptom you can see it coming from a process of overall improvement rather than of deterioration you are well on the way.

Like anything truly worthwhile, it can take some time to get really well. As you use herbs along with improved nutrition and exercise, your body will heave a sigh of relief and begin to look at its deeper layers of imbalance! In the naturopathic tradition people are expected to experience 'healing crises' as they have symptoms in reverse order and go back through their history of illness. Although the reversal occurs in all forms of natural healing - it's like peeling off the old layers and uncovering a fresh healthy person underneath - you do not have to experience healing crises in such a raw form. By following the recommendations for diet, supplements, and other aids to healing, the more uncomfortable symptoms are often avoided. By using the different herbal combinations as the appropriate symptoms come to the fore, the course of overall healing is maintained while the area of symptoms can be dealt with.

Very few people can jump in at the deep end and change their life completely in order to feel healthier. Although I would say health affects every aspect of our life for better or worse, I know that I would not have listened to that twenty years ago. If you are standing on the edge of the pool wondering whether to test the water, you can be reassured that herbs are not habit forming and you can use them without committing yourself to plunging up to your ears in health-mania!

# Summarising

This approach to healing is based firmly on the existing knowledge about herbs and natural healing methods. But it looks at the process with a new way of understanding. All the elements of this view have been discovered by others and the underlying logic has been presented as Trialectics by Oscar Ichazo (26)(a logic that reflects reality much more successfully than dialectics or formal logic). So I do not claim originality. But I do claim that this view works. As soon as you have it, your health and whole life will change for the better. Not because this is the latest slogan or sales pitch, but because it works.

Let us look again at the elements:

1. We are responsible for our own body, our degree of health.
2. Sources of knowledge of the body must include feeling as well as science.
3. To understand the body, health etc., there are three types of reasoning, analysis, comparison and empathy.
4. The body consists of matter and energy in different levels of organisation - atoms, cells, tissues, systems, emotions, mind, spirit.
5. Consciousness can awaken to the whole body, or it can be locked in illusion.
6. There are correlations between the different levels of the body, between thoughts, emotions and systems, for example.
7. There are important balances within each level of the body and harmonies between levels.
8. Health involves balance and harmony, given that the body is continually adapting and evolving. There is a process of health and a state of transcendent health.
9. When we get involved in fighting or destroying illness the balance of health is always at a lower level. This is the problem of medicine, drugs and surgery.
10. Some agents of imbalance are toxicity, stress and malnutrition. These external agents relate directly to our internal state.
11. The body has inbuilt ways of adapting to imbalances.
12. Symptoms are the expression of the body's attempts to deal with imbalance by adapting.
13. As natural healers, herbs encourage the body to adapt,

throw off toxicity, manage stress and improve nutrition while aiding specific organs or tissues.

14. The efficacy of herbs is recognised in a clinical/scientific tradition and an intuitive tradition.

15. Herbs work as foods, because of drug-like effects, 'homoeopathic' pattern effects and because of a vibrational affinity with the body.

16. The method of developing intuitive understanding of herbs involves understanding ourselves and our bodies as well as plants.

17. We can get well at our own pace, and using herbs we can uncover a healthier self.

*References:*
1. *P. Rawson, L. Legeza. Tao. Thames & Hudson. 1973.*
2. *O. Ichazo. Between Metaphysics and Protoanalysis.*
   *Arica Institute Press. 1982.*
3. *W. Heisenberg. In Physics and Beyond. Harper & Row. 1971.*
4. *C. Darwin. The Origin of Species. Penguin.*
5. *J. Bleibtrau. The Parable of the Beast. Gollancz. 1968.*
6. *F. Mann. Acupuncture. Pan. 1971.*
7. *G. Vithoulkas. The Science of Homoeopathy. Grove Press. 1980.*
8. *W. Evans-Wentz Ed. The Tibetan Book of the Dead. OUP. 1960.*
9. *O. Ichazo. Levels of Consciousness, Domains of Consciousness. Trainings of Arica Inst. Inc. For more information on Arica contact the author.*
10. *O. Ichazo. Doors of Compensation Training. Arica Institute Inc.*
11. *O. Ichazo. Op. cit. 2.*
12. *J.I. Rodale. The Complete Book of Minerals for Health. Rodale Books. 1976.*
13. *C. Pfeiffer. Mental and Elemental Nutrients. Keats. 1975.*
14. *H. Selye. The Stress of Life. McGraw Hill. 1976.*
15. *O. Ichazo. Chua Ka Massage.*
16. *C. Gerras. The Complete Book of Vitamins. Rodale. 1977.*
17. *W.H. Lewis, M.P.F. Lewis. Medical Botany.*
   *John Wiley & Sons. 1977.*
18. *B.N. Ames. Dietary Carcinogens and Anticarcinogens.*
   *Science 221. 1983.*
19. *J. Harvey, D.G.C. Jones. Brit. Med. J. 282. 1981.*
20. *Mrs. M. Grieve. A Modern Herbal. Peregrine. 1976.*
21. *C. Ponc. Alchemy. N. Atlantic Books. 1983.*
22. *N. Weeks. The Medical Discoveries of Edward Bach, Physician.*
   *C.W. Daniel.*
23. *G. Zukav. The Dancing Wu Li Masters. Bantam. 1979.*
24. *D.V. Tansley. Subtle Body. Thames & Hudson. 1977.*
25. *F. Mann. op. cit. 6.*
26. *O. Ichazo. op cit. 2.*

Part Two

---

# Three Stories of Healing Through Herbs

# The Source of the Stories

Having worked with these herbs over a number of years I have inevitably been in contact with a number of people who have undertaken courses of herbal healing, from 'one-off' attempts to deal with symptoms to extended periods of deep healing.

Rather than give a large number of clinical accounts, it seems more informative and entertaining to give three composite stories which are in some ways typical of people's approaches and attitudes to healing themselves the herbal way.

**Jane**

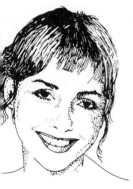

Jane has just discovered that she is pregnant. She is very pleased and excited. It adds another facet to a full life and will mean some adjustments. But Jane is used to adjusting.

Two years ago she was depressed, overweight, had irregular and very painful menstruation and found it impossible to do anything but handle her exacting job in buying and selling fabrics. By 26 she had used her mind a great deal at school, university, in business and in the struggles to get work, and the right kind of job. She had been through a lot of emotional learning through relationships, disappointments and the effects of her independence and desire for freedom. At school she had been a fair athelete, but apart from some attempts at dieting for weight loss, had to admit since then she had ignored her body. A vicious circle had begun of feeling bored and limited, eating, feeling guilty and unattractive and therefore not able to enjoy herself.

At this point Jane was ready to try something different, and she decided that her body needed attention first. She started to look at her appetite, began using Herbal A, ginseng and fenugreek, one before each meal. She slowly started to substitute raw vegetables and salads with fish for the habitual hamburger, bun, chips and ketchup, and ate fruit between meals instead of chocolate biscuits. This was a lot different from her usual diets during which she felt listless, angry and exhausted. She felt she was getting 'too calm' and needed a way of boosting energy and burning off some of the extra 'tyres'.

We worked out a programme which concentrated less on counting calories than on eating for maximum health. She would have a good breakfast of yoghurt, fruit salad and/or non sugared muesli with fresh juice. She took seeds, nuts and a little dried fruit to work and had a salad, crudites vegetables and cheese dip or just fresh fruit for lunch. She would drink plenty of water, no coffee or sugared drinks, a little weak tea, an occasional glass of wine in the evening. The evening meal was again mainly raw vegetables or a Greek salad or sprouted beans and seeds, with cauliflower cheese, fish, liver, brown rice with lentils, poached eggs, or baked potato with low-salt cheese. She worked at making her food interesting and quickly found alternative tastes to compensate for a ban on sugar and salt.

To make sure her metabolism was fast and efficient, and to reduce water retention and cellulite, Jane used six special kelp tablets (kelp, dandelion and alfalfa) daily over the first month, reducing to four for six months. She also used a strong multivitamin/mineral with a high B complex for energy and conversion of fats with extra lecithin for fat transport in the body.

The first thing she noticed was that she started getting up with enthusiasm for the day and coming home wanting to see people instead of lie and doze. Over the next six months there was a consistent weight loss, return of positive attitude to her body and more energy.

The only times when this progress seemed to reverse completely was just before and during menstruation. Jane became depressed, touchy and slightly bloated. She was ready after a few months of noticing the difference from her new self, to do something about it. She had found a man she wanted to have a family with and really wanted to sort out the whole of her female chemistry, regularising periods, sorting out odd aches in the uterus area, getting rid of a tendency to thrush and making sure she was ready for pregnancy.

So she began a course of Herbal F, Female Tonic. She felt that the liquorice was cleansing and healing her while black cohosh and mistletoe were helping with menstruation and Raspberry leaf preparing her for pregnancy. Though this is a simplistic view there is no doubt that her strong feeling for the mixture helped her body use it. She had three tablets a day for four months, had a month's break and continued in the same pattern up to now. She also used extra B6 100mg and magnesium 400mg to manage particularly bad PMT. She reduced that dosage to almost nil after a year.

As we all do, Jane went off her diet after two months. She was starting to get depressed and put on weight when she heard about the effect of a bad diet on the colon - the build up of sticky and encrusted mucus leading to mucus and toxins in the whole body. This 'horror story' led her to fast on fruit for a week and commence cleansing. She used four each of Herbal G and D daily to clear through the intestines and also cleanse blood, liver, kidneys and whole body. After a month, she was feeling lighter and cleaner, she could think more clearly and she no longer needed a deodorant! She repeated this nine months later and will do it again a few months after the baby is born.

Jane has found that she can affect her thinking and feeling as well as her weight, energy and health, by using herbs along with diet. She knows that she can go on progressing and improving - and that she doesn't have to be exhausted and enslaved by childbirth, her job, her marriage or her expectations of ageing. Much more than a knowledge of herbs, this confidence about the pattern of health throughout life is the key to success in enjoying and fulfilling herself.

She will use Herbal F to condition the glands and muscles for delivery, and will start on Herbal M (fennel and fenugreek), the 'mothers' combination to maintain her water balance, improve the condition of her breasts and help her to get the most out of breastfeeding. She knows that nutrition for her child is directly dependent on her own nutrition, not only when she is breastfeeding, but afterwards when she chooses real food rather than processed 'babyfood' and when she uses diluted herbs, vitamins, minerals and other natural aids to balance childhood ailments.

## Roger

Roger is a vigorous and lively man of 40 who has spent the last seven years travelling and living in the exciting world of theatre. His creativity is his major preoccupation and he uses it in intensive, exhausting bursts in his job as a set designer.

He had the usual childhood and adolescent illnesses and some debilitating infections during his 20's like German measles and glandular fever. He had conventional drug treatment. In the last five years he became interested in health

45

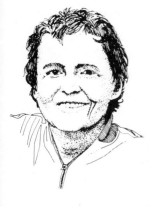

foods, tried various natural treatments for his regular colds and generally avoided drugs when he became exhausted.

When I saw him he was suffering from a miserable bout of flu which started his body aching as soon as he had tied up the last production. He felt too ill to eat, which was just as well, and we worked out the fruits and juices he likes plus a simple vegetable gruel which he or his girlfriend could prepare in the evening. He took 5 grams of vitamin C, 25,000iu of A and a multivitamin/mineral daily plus 2 tablets of Infection and Fever, Herbal I, three times a day. He was more comfortable that night and in two days he was not only better, but he said that he felt quite restored in energy. After taking the tablets for three more days he felt 'too well to be taking anything' and stopped using herbs or supplements.

The next time I saw him, after several months, he complained that his current project was keeping him awake at night and making him tired and snappish in the mornings. He had taken a sleeping tablet once but found that he felt worse. Herbal Sleep combination starting 2 tablets in the evening and 2 at night helped to relax him and he was able to sleep well providing he did not get too over-excited. After the project finished he used them occasionally when he needed help to relax. Although once he used eight tablets on a particularly awful night, he noticed no after effects. To help his body to get going and operate more smoothly, he used two Herbal T tablets in the morning, and sometimes two after lunch. He found that they quickly eliminated the drowsiness due to too much food and drink.

Roger's body was beginning to surface after years of struggling with run down glandular and immune systems and the limiting effects of toxic drug residues. Feeling better, he wanted to maintain progress by improving his diet and using vitamins and minerals. But he wasn't yet ready to be really consistent in his approach to self-healing.

In the winter of that first year he got his usual colds. With the second one he took no aspirins but kept warm and took vitamins A and C and two Herbal C (Cold and Congestion combination) tablets three times a day. As soon as the symptoms went, he cut down to two and then one tablet a day.

This was really a major turning point. He was able to throw off some old poisons along with the colds and mucus and felt considerably clearer afterwards.

He decided in the spring that he would start to clean up

his body. So he began with one day drinking only juices, three days on unlimited fruit, and three days on fish, yoghurt, vegetables, fruit, and water, juices and herb teas. He took two Herbal D, Detoxifying and Cleansing, tablets three times a day and the vitamins and minerals recommended. During the detoxification process he said he sometimes felt terrible. I advised him to drink spring water and lemon juice and lie down for a while, feel the discomforts in his body and let his mind follow whatever thoughts came up. One vivid memory was of lying in bed with chickenpox, hearing his mother talking with the doctor and imagining that he would die of itching. The day after this during the course of the fast his skin seemed to him much smoother and cleaner. By the end of the detoxification process some old poisons had been removed and some of the recent medical drugs, alcohol and excess sugar and salt had been neutralised and removed, leaving him feeling clearer in body and mind and more energetic.

As Roger was busier now than ever before he wanted to find a way to maintain his energy. He realised that he was not nearly at the end of his healing process, but wasn't sure quite how to proceed. In the end he decided on a month's trial of each of the combinations Anti Stress, K special kelp and T Tonic and Stimulant.

He found the ginseng effect quite subtle and it was only at the end of the month when he looked back, that he realised that he had more resistance to stress, he could work longer without reaching exhaustion. He found with kelp that he dropped a little excess weight quite quickly but the effect after a month was not so marked. Then he had a month on Herbal T. This really seemed quite immediate in terms of effect on waking up his body, but didn't have the long term resistance-building of ginseng. So he decided that Anti Stress was the one to take regular courses of, with Herbal T as a back-up.

It was difficult to persuade Roger to rest properly and he had a bout of flu later in that year. He cleared up quite well using Herbal I, but it made him think about taking detoxification and slow natural rebalancing quite seriously. During a further exhausting trip he developed conjunctivitis, another sign of throwing off old poisons, this time less bothersome than a cold. He used Herbal E, Eye Tonic to help clear this condition and his eyes.

He now quite regularly undertakes a week of cleansing

using Herbal D and every other three months takes a course of Triple Ginseng. He uses S and T when there are difficulties sleeping and waking. He is quite optimistic now about having no further colds, flu or other infections, but recognises that he can bring them on through exhaustion. He finds it easier now to control excesses in his diet and uses vitamins and other supplements along with herbs. He does have periods when he forgets or gives up on his programme, but ultimately he recognises that he can be more efficient and creative when he is naturally 'high' than when this comes from straining himself or using drug medicine to maintain only a minimum level of health.

## Florence

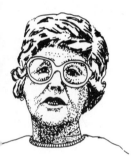

Florence is 65, a retired teacher who found it more and more difficult to have the active retirement she dreamed of. Her arthritis got much worse when her husband died five years ago and she had pain in her hips, knees, hands and feet. She had aspirin treatment but gave it up when it ruined her digestion and her sleep, and then had occasional sleeping tablets.

Although Florence tried to exercise daily, and this showed her will to stay mobile, she was very resistant to changing her diet in any way. Only that day, she said, she had heard a doctor on the radio say that arthritis is nothing to do with diet! But she didn't want surgery or the doubtful cortisone or gold injection treatment and was looking for something to give her relief without side effects.

At the beginning she just took three Herbal R, Rheumatism and Arthritis, tablets daily. Over the course of two weeks there was slight improvement in the pain and she had been out shopping more than in the last six months.

We explained how sugar is one of the major stressors which sets up the glandular imbalance underlying arthritis. She grudgingly agreed to change her diet if we could suggest something for her 'nerves' and to help her to sleep. She quite rightly pointed out that her tension, lack of sleep and use of sleeping pills were stress factors.

Maintaining the Herbal R, she cut her sugar down to one home made cake a day, cut out most salty, frozen and tinned food and made valient efforts to consume salads and fruit. She actually found that a juicer and a set of sprouting jars became more important than the cooker. At the same time she had two Herbal H (Head and Nerves) tablets in the morning to reduce her anxiety and tension about the day, and two Herbal S (Sleep) tablets an hour before sleeping. She also had a high B complex multi with B5 500mg and vitamin C 1000mg in the morning and five bonemeal tablets in the evening.

A month on this rigorous programme showed an amazing improvement. Florence looked ten years younger. She had lost the lines of tension and tiredness on her face and greeted us with enthusiasm and was full of plans for the day. She was sleeping much better and had trailed off the use of sleeping tablets.

But shortly after, she suffered pain, a sleepless night and a sudden loss of faith. She had been moving too fast. During the next three months she found more of a comfortable balance in her eating and took her herbs and supplements only when she felt like it.

She asked for advice again when she had high blood pressure diagnosed. She had been told to take drugs to control it, but wanted to find a more natural way. Garlic, cayenne and kelp we said - Herbal B. Also we reminded her that salt was one of the no-no's in her diet, and that it was primarily responsible for hypertension. We also described a journey down her blood vessels and linked to that deterioration and 'furring up' in joints and muscles causing arthritis and rheumatism. She used three a day for about three months and we heard no more from her for six months.

Florence planned a holiday in the summer. She wanted to walk with her friend. She had real motivation to get fit. She went back on her diet and vitamins and minerals. She used four Herbal R a day, occasionally Herbal S for sleep and no longer needed H or B; she doubled her B5 and C dosage. After three months she was walking a mile daily, doing exercises for fingers and toes and feeling much less pain. She enjoyed her holiday.

If Florence found the motivation to live fully, which others find at her age and much older, she would be able to undo the years of neglect and unbalanced treatment which led to arthritis. On the way she would find other areas and imbalances claiming attention. For instance her tissues are quite hardened by tension and toxicity which would come out in stages, and her digestive system is geared to clogging mucus, inadequate enzymes and the wrong bacteria. The way back to health is layer by layer, but the feeling of fulfilment increases with each layer stripped.

Part Three

---

# Herbal Combinations and Healing Programmes

# Introduction

**Where do the Combinations come from?**

The herbs used in the 15 Combinations all have an ancient history of use. We have now worked with them for ten years and regard them with increasing respect as we learn more about their application. Some of them were suggested through a medium who worked very successfully in herbalism and natural healing, Marshall Lever. They are so gentle that they can be used regularly as preventives for very minor imbalances, or to tune up your body. But they are also effective aids to healing more serious conditions and illnesses. It is recommended that serious or prolonged conditions are discussed with your practitioner.

**The Body**

In each chapter on herbs you will find a description of the body. To be able to see how to use the herbs, you will need more than a list of diseases and illnesses they are designed to work with. Understanding the state of the body is vital to healing because it allows you to harmonise with the healing process. The BODY sections are designed to help you focus attention rather than gather facts, so it helps to read them with the questions in mind, 'how does this apply to me?' or 'is this what is happening in my body?' You should also refer to the drawings and use them both to tune in to what is happening and to visualise your return to full health.

**The Herbs**

These healing herbs are inclined to be strong-tasting. Also it is best to take them whole. For these reasons we do not recommend teas, tisanes or other extractions as highly. They are best taken ground and mixed with honey, or in capsules or tablets prepared without changing the herbs and with only natural tableting agents.

In herbal lore many of the herbs have traditional uses and sometimes spectacular cures are a matter of historical record. Herbs also have inter-relationships, and by combining them we may amplify certain effects. Golden seal is a well known amplifier of other herbs' effects, particularly on body membranes, possibly because it carries other herbal components along with its penetrating oils. Cayenne has a similar effect. But in each combination there is an area of

53

interaction where the effect of the whole is greater than the sum of the parts. These effects are summarised under the heading THE COMBINATION.

The section on THE HERBS gives more background on each of the herbs individually. The pictures of the herbs can be used to give an impression of their particular energy.

Lastly in each chapter you will find a brief note on THE MIXTURE. This is for the benefit of those who do not have the pleasure of grinding and combining their herbs. It gives an impression of the overall feel of the combination, particularly with reference to the elements of earth, water, fire and air. This is not strictly using a theory of the elements but simply a way of reminding our senses of the similarities and associations they might make if experiencing the herbs 'in the raw'.

## Nutrition

You will find that the effects of herbs on your health is less if diet includes salt, sugar, preservatives, additives and the 'foods' which have been processed until they are empty of nutrients.

A more thorough guide to diet is to be found in other of our publications. But given here are some of the more important guidelines. You can build a complete programme of herbs, foods and supplements along these guidelines.

## Supplements

A maintenance programme of supplements ensures that all your basic reqirements for vitamins and minerals is covered. At minimum we suggest 1 multivitamin containing vitamin A, the full B complex, vitamins D and E, 1 gram of vitamin C and a full multimineral. Details of daily amounts can be found on page152.

Many imbalances are due to long term deficiencies of particular nutrients. Deficiences may arise through mother's deficiences, genetic difficulties in uptake or use, and early exposure to stress. These prenatal factors can dispose people to very high needs for certain nutrients. For instance some people need several grams of niacin, vitamin B3, to prevent schizophrenic symptoms, whereas normal requirements are in tens, and units of milligrams.

Later, drugs may wipe out vitamins or minerals, or cause structural or chemical damage which supplements can help repair. Our diet may simply have lacked essential nutrients, or we may have used up supplies by overeating, say, sugar. Though we can normally simply replace the nutrient, sometimes the body by-passes the normal biochemical pathways. Then it must be saturated by the missing nutrient to help the normal pathway to be found again. This approach is known as orthomolecular therapy or megavitamin therapy and is harmonious with herbs.

**Other Aids**

In a process of healing, mental and emotional life must be considered. In the first place, an illness may be the expression of mental or emotional imbalance, and then physical treatment alone will not be effective.

Secondly, there is no physical symptom that does not have correspondences in emotions and mind. For instance, difficulty in the liver's ability to sort out food substances may parallel difficulty in organising your life or feeling secure with your arrangements.

You may find yourself having to work on all the realms at once, or you may find that as you heal your body, thoughts, memories and feelings come to you 'out of the blue'. So while working with herbs, it is recommended that you develop a method for mind and emotions, while developing the spiritual realm too.

Start with relaxation, and becoming aware of your breathing. Sit comfortably or lie down and relax your body methodically - face, head, neck, shoulders, arms, torso, back, belly, buttocks, legs, feet. Allowing your abdominal muscles to relax, breathe into the deepest point in the belly.

Gradually fill your lungs from the bottom to the top, allowing the abdomen and the whole ribcage to expand completely. Breathe out from the top, emptying the last of your breath from the very bottom. When you reach a stage of comfort and relaxation, your mind fills with thoughts and images. Every time you get caught up in these, your breathing changes, becomes shallow and irregular, and you lose relaxation.

Think of an area of your life which causes you difficulty. You may feel hot and uncomfortable when you hit the 'target' area. Focus on this particular incident which provoked this emotion and picture it exactly as it happened. When you feel emotional again, return to relaxation and start seeing the incident again imagining that you are a completely impartial observer. Repeat the process until you can see the incident clearly from an objective, uninvolved viewpoint. At that point you may realise you felt strongly because you hold a belief, or a whole system of beliefs, that you do not necessarily need. For instance, you might have felt unloved because your friend did not say 'Good morning'. When you can see what happened and how you felt, you might realise that you held on to a belief in 'good manners' which does not fit with the realities of friendship. It helps to ask yourself when you felt this way before, and before that, and so on. When you have identified irrational and unnecessary belief areas, and perhaps traced them back to their origin, you can let them go with relief, and hopefully will remember not to get trapped by them next time.

Negative feelings are held in the subconscious mind, which is a very mechanical part of our nature, susceptible to gentle positive guidance. Remember that reality does not follow directly on any affirmation you care to make, but as perception and thought processes evolve, our reality changes too. Do not use affirmation as self-hypnosis, since all methods which force change are out of step with natural healing. The point is to become aware of thoughts and feelings and to remind yourself of the real transcendental truths.

Visualisation can be used to accelerate physical healing. By picturing the body changing and healing we dissolve mental barriers to the healing process. You could visualise your digestive system working in perfect balance and imagine that you are getting the best possible nutrition from your food. By imagining consistently a team of fairies and pixies cleansing and removing diseased cells a woman speeded her complete recovery from cancer of the cervix.

Healing is always a matter of being in tune with our Creator's will. Everything else is heading for illusion and unhappiness.

Tension and structural imbalance can be worked on in a number of ways. Exercise, such as walking, swimming, running or yoga is very important, and should always be done with attention to breathing so that further tension is not built up. Natural physical therapies such as Alexander Technique, Chua Ka, Cranial Osteopathy, Feldenkrais, Massage, Reflexology, Rolfing and Touch for Health, can be great aids at the right time. Two highly recommended therapeutic exercises are T'ai Chi and Arica Psychocalisthenics®.

There is now an enormous range of natural therapies available, all of which offer a great deal. Different people are attuned to different therapies, so it isn't possible to give guarantees of success, and as most of them would point out, it is the patient who cures him or herself. Having experienced many I would say that they each have a focus and you can heal yourself from many complementary angles. Having a map of your body and the way it works is the best background to choosing wisely which therapies might help you.

So, equipped with a battery of aids to health, you are ready to make full use of the wonderful herbal combinations which form the central dynamic point of a complete method of natural healing.

# Herbal A  *Appetite and Digestion*

As well as for health promotion useful in these conditions:

Anorexia, appetite disturbances, digestion - incomplete, slow, nervous, painful or poor assimilation, diarrhoea, flatulence, hypo and hyper-glycemia, nausea, obesity, ulcers, vomiting. Can't take in ideas or information. Can't assimilate emotional situations.
*(For any serious or lasting condition consult your practitioner)*

**Ginseng**    root   *Panax ginseng*
**Fenugreek**  seed   *Trigonella foenum -graecum*

As powder up to 1 gram daily, or 200mg of each, per tablet, 1-5 daily. Courses of no longer than 6 months. Women who suffer heavy menstrual bleeding should be cautious about ginseng. Also if this combination makes you feel over-energised you should use it with caution.

## The Body
Small intestine wall

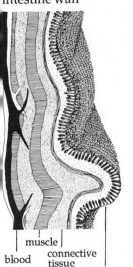

muscle
blood and lymph supply
connective tissue
secretory and absorptive skin

The whole of the digestive system is, in a sense, outside the body as it continues the skin barrier, somewhat like a doughnut! You could picture the inner surface as a soft towelling exposed to food mixed with digestive juices.

The first part of the system, up to the stomach is mainly concerned with secreting digestive enzymes to begin protein, starch and fat digestion. The stomach is a muscular bag producing helpful acid and mucus which aid digestion, but it, like the mouth is a sensitive area responding to types of food and to the suitability of the time, place and emotional state for eating. In times of stress, the adrenal hormones shut down activity here, reducing appetite and calling up reserves of protein from the stomach walls - hence stress ulcers.

Food is released gradually from the stomach into the duodenum, where it mixes with bile from the liver and gall bladder, used for fat digestion, and enzymes-plus-alkali from the pancreas, to further break down proteins, starches and fats. The pancreas is very much affected by sugar in the diet, and the liver by fats.

In the small intestine, each frond of the "towel", or villus, has a single line of absorbing and secreting cells, and it is here that the final breakdown of food should occur, and active absorption into lymph and blood vessels takes place. Hormones and nerve signals help to control the vast amount of absorption, and the muscles controlling the passage of contents through the small intestine must be maintained in good condition.

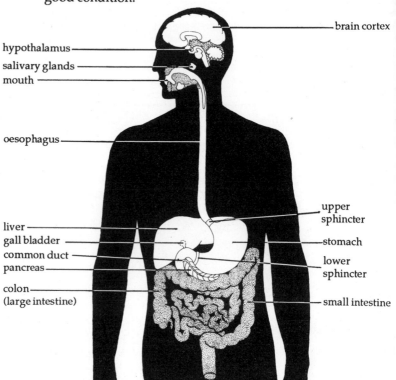

In the large intestine the contents are concentrated, water and other nutrients absorbed, and wastes eliminated, all with the help of a bacterial "garden". We may develop constipation, putrefaction, diarrhoea and so on, especially if we have the balance of digestion wrong further back in the system.

The balance of nerves and hormones communicating throughout the digestive system tells us about our food needs, together with the hypothalamus brain centre which tells us about blood contents. Appetite is very liable to get mixed up with the way we feel and think, and is often confused by our habits and addictions. We can unlearn some of these primitive reactions by improving and becoming more conscious of the effects of our nerves and glands on appetite.

# The Herbs
## *Ginseng*

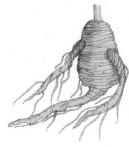

Ginseng is arousing enormous interest in the West following centuries of use in the East and recent scientific interest in the U.S.S.R

It reduces overstimulation of the adrenal cortex (used in the stress reaction) and gives us a calm and good blood supply to the system for proper digestion. It contains a spectrum of substances known as adaptogens, which gently bring the glandular system back to homeostatic balance. The nervous system is tranquillised, rebuilt and rebalanced, reducing depression and restoring appetite control. It has been demonstrated scientifically in animals that ginseng raises hormone levels to cope with stress while blood sugar is not raised [1], and it can raise the production of insulin in the pancreas of diabetic animals [2].

The American Indians used it to prevent nausea and vomiting, and its use as a stomachic is well recognised in European herbals. It conditions the digestive glands throughout the system giving an adequate flow of digestive juices. A ginseng extract fed to animals in an experiment helped to emulsify fats and cholesterol for better digestion, and stimulated the absorption of fat-soluble vitamins A and E [3].

Muscular tone is restored in the whole digestive system. Ginseng stimulates cellular metabolism, helping to rebuild muscle, blood and tissues, and aiding the successful conversion of food in the body.

Perhaps more than any other herb, ginseng acts gently and cumulatively and is often best taken over several months.

## *Fenugreek*

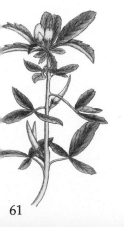

Fenugreek was used by the ancient Egyptians and is famous for its anti-inflammation properties. It produces a strong mucilage which is very comforting for stomach and intestines and soothes nerves, glands and soft membranes. It is good for mouth and stomach ulcers.

Fenugreek contains B vitamins 1, 2 and 3, and aids in their absorption. This directly benefits nerves, enzyme production and metabolic processes involving proteins, fats and carbohydrates. It contains another B complex vitamin, choline, which aids the transport and breakdown of cholesterol into bile, cleansing the liver and blood and helping the digestion of fats.

Fenugreek is particularly noted for its effect on the pancreas, improving enzyme production and helping with the balance of sugar in the blood. It is a traditional aid for diabetes in the Middle East, and is thought to inhibit over-production of the blood sugar raising hormone, glucagon, as well as normalising insulin production (4). It stimulates the flow of digestive juices, liquid food substances and all liquid processes in the body.

## The Mixture

The mixture is soft light brown and smells like warm earth. Ginseng supplies the warmth, but mainly the balancing of earth. Fenugreek has a more watery energy together with warm penetrating oils which are carried throughout the body.

## Nutrition

Vegetables and fruit should form the greatest percentage of diet. Avoid excessive amounts of sugar, salt, alcohol or other drugs which are disruptive to the digestion and the whole metabolism. Fried and oily foods are also difficult to digest, as are some food combinations like protein/fruit or protein/starch. Aluminium from foil, cooking pots and added to food or drinking water is a great source of digestive disorder and flatulence since the metal affects the pancreas and its alkaline juices and poisons the body. Fresh vegetable juice, fruit juice and lightly cooked soups are good liquid nutrition, and sprouted seeds and grains make good solid foods for sensitive stomachs. Blood sugar can become more balanced if the food source is broken down into sugars slowly. Whole grains, especially oats and millet, South American quinoa, rice and lentils, beans, pulses and buckwheat are excellent sources of protein, starches, sugars and fibre. They have been used successfully in bringing blood sugar and appetite problems under control.

## Supplements

In addition to a full complement of vitamins and minerals, for appetite disturbances you may find these useful:

Vitamin B complex (75mg major B's),
Zinc (50mg chelated). Zinc deficiency is a major cause of anorexia.
Digestive enzymes mixture with lactase if there are milk
    digestion problems.
Papaya enzymes.
Pancreatin 1000mg
Chromium 200mcg
    (preferably GTF Chromium)

*For ulcers:*
Vitamin A (25-75,000iu for 1 month)
Vitamin C (as magnesium ascorbate 2000mg)
Vitamin E (400-1000iu providing no heart complaint)
Zinc (50mg chelated)
L-glutamine (1000mg)

## Other Aids

Whenever you eat, picture the food supplying energy and the right molecules through the digestive system wall, via blood and lymph, to all parts of the body. Say to yourself "with every meal my appetite is balanced and my body receives all it needs in comfort."

Massage of the abdomen, reflexology and Touch for Health techniques are very useful for releasing tensions around the digestive organs. The digestive system is very very prone to emotionally based tensions and the breathing and relaxation technique is very applicable.

I have found the herbal combination useful for people who need a persistent gentle treatment. A woman with ' delicate digestion' who jumped from extreme loss of appetite to occasional binges found that using this combination alone for two weeks allowed her to start taking regular supplements. Using extra B vitamins and zinc and the herbs for three months brought her towards a much more stable state. She found that she could recognise when she was going toward the extremes again and was able to control this tendency by including herbs and supplements in her diet.

*References:*
1. *S. Hiai et al. Chem. Pharm. Bull. 31. 1983.*
2. *I. Waki et al. J. Pharm. Dyn. 5. 1982.*
3. *I. Waki. Ibid.*
4. *A. Nelson. Medical Botany. Livingstone. 1951.*

# Herbal B    *Blood and Circulation*

As well as for health promotion, useful in these conditions:

Angina pectoris, arteriosclerosis, atherosclerosis, broken capillaries, high blood pressure, bruising, chilblains, coronary thrombosis, embolism, hypertension, heart disease, poor circulation, stroke, varicose veins.

*(For any serious or lasting condition consult your practitioner)*

| | | |
|---|---|---|
| **Garlic** | bulb | *Allium sativum* |
| **Cayenne** | fruit | *Capsicum minimum* |
| **Kelp** | herb (seaweed) | *Fucus vesiculosis* |

As powder 3/4 gram of each daily, or 150mg of each, per tablet, 1-5 tablets daily.

## The Body

The blood within a vessel contains many large red and white corpuscles, together with platelets, fat droplets and a thick soup of disolved nutrients, the plasma. This viscous mixture flows down the arteries at great speed, and returns under pressure through capillaries and veins to the heart. The vessel walls, therefore, must be in excellent health to allow free flow of blood.

As any plumber would know, this is a difficult order, and problems with blood vessels are almost epidemic in the West. The artery wall commonly loses flexibility and suffers damage because of deficiencies of essential vitamins and minerals. Free fatty acids from refined oil, margarine and fried food, or oxidising chemicals from pollutants in food or air may attack the inner lining. Wastes and over-concentrations of natural substances like cholesterol and calcium gather around these weaknesses causing plaque. The consequent narrowing of the arteries and loss of flexibility form the basis of many heart and circulation problems. When the walls of capillaries and veins are weakened, bruising, varicose veins, strokes and "bad circulation" may result. Kidneys are affected, in turn changing blood composition and concentration.

Adrenal, pituitary, thyroid and parathyroid glands control blood levels of cholesterol, calcium, other minerals and nutrients, and directly affect heart rate, arterial flow and metabolic rate. A high salt intake will affect the kidneys and adrenals and is a well-recognised cause of hypertension.

The autonomic nervous system controls the amount and flow of blood through heart, spleen and arteries. These systems must work in harmony for circulatory health and any healing must take into account the whole pattern.

The heart's muscular tissue, connective tissue, linings and valves must have a correct supply of vitamins, minerals and nutrients, or the heart will degenerate. Any such symptoms signify a need to heal the whole circulatory system.

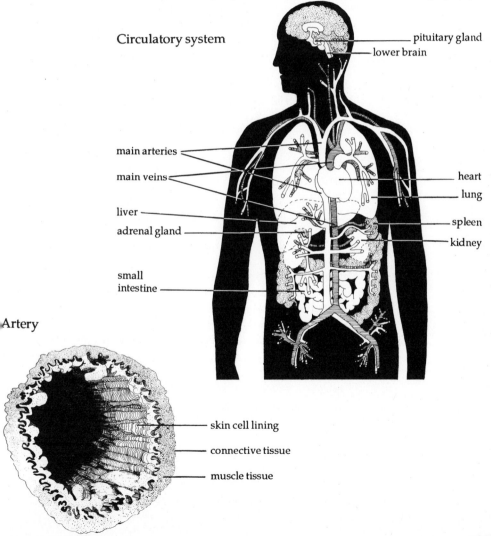

Circulatory system

pituitary gland

lower brain

main arteries

main veins

heart

lung

liver

spleen

adrenal gland

kidney

small intestine

Artery

skin cell lining

connective tissue

muscle tissue

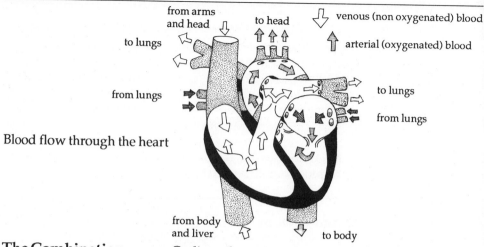

from arms and head

to head

venous (non oxygenated) blood

arterial (oxygenated) blood

to lungs

from lungs

to lungs

from lungs

Blood flow through the heart

from body and liver

to body

**The Combination**    Garlic and cayenne are antiseptic and very powerful cleansers of the circulatory system. All three cleanse and tone the digestive system and encourage supply of foods, vitamins, minerals and trace elements, to the blood. Cayenne stimulates, kelp tones the glandular system, keeping circulation free of stress-induced imbalances. Garlic calms, cayenne stimulates, kelp nourishes the nervous system for correct regulation of blood flow.

**The Herbs**
*Garlic*

That garlic prevents heart disease has been known for centuries. It is one of the most widely used herbs in Europe and the East and is famous for its protective and cleansing properties. It has long been used for atherosclerosis and high blood pressure and many associated problems.

In a series of experiments, high cholesterol and fat levels have been produced in animals by feeding them on a high sugar, or a high fat diet. In both cases, a large dose of the pungent, sulphurous allyl oils of garlic completely nullified the effects of the diets [1]. Garlic not only reduces the body's production of cholesterol, it also cuts down the dangerous LDL cholesterol, while leaving the essential HDL cholesterol, and so is most beneficial for atherosclerosis [2]. It helps to break down the layers of plaque and rejuvenate artery tissues. It seems to reduce the likelihood of clotting, thrombosis, by decreasing the clumping of blood platelets, and in some people has a normalising effect on blood pressure [3].

Garlic contains and aids the assimilation of vitamins, A, B,C, minerals including iodine, phosphorus and sulphur. It contains hormone-like substances and tones thyroid glands

*Cayenne*

Taken on the tongue, or rubbed on the skin, cayenne makes the area hot and red. It does this by acting on the autonomic nerves to dilate the small peripheral blood vessels. But it does not irritate the skin surface, and in fact the irritating histamine response is abolished by cayenne (4). So it stimulates and warms the whole circulatory system, revitalising lethargic areas, strengthening the heart and arteries, and opening the smaller blood vessels. It stimulates repair of damaged capillaries, and the walls of the heart, arteries and veins. It soothes the cells lining the lungs after exposure to cigarette smoke and other irritants (5).

Containing and aiding the absorption of vitamins A and C, minerals sulphur, phosphorus, magnesium, calcium and iron, cayenne balances the glands, catalyses the effects of other herbs and helps in the cleansing and removal of plaque. Cayenne has been shown to give "significant protection against cardiovascular disease by lowering blood cholesterol and inhibiting the formation of thrombi (blood clots)" (6).

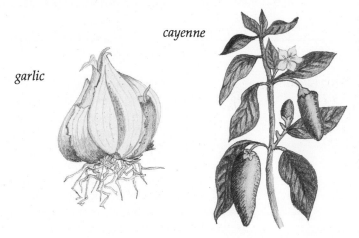

*cayenne*

*garlic*

*Kelp*

Kelp is a good cleanser, its alginic acid helping to remove heavy metals, such as cadmium, which can damage the heart. Kelp contains perhaps the widest spectrum of vitamins and minerals amongst the herbs, particularly trace elements. This makes it valuable for all metabolic processes, particularly glandular and nervous, and provides some necessary nutrients for rebuilding blood vessels. Its potassium helps to balance salt excess, reducing adrenal stimulation and hypertension, and provides the heart with one of the most essential minerals for its contractions. Through its iodine content it conditions the thyroid gland, reducing fats and the tendency to obesity - a major risk factor for circulatory disease.

*kelp*

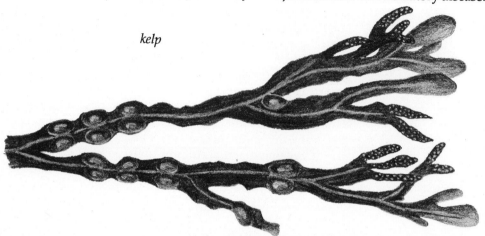

**The Mixture**

The mixture smells and tastes powerfully fiery, allowing it to penetrate and cleanse through all the tissues. The watery nature of garlic and kelp open a flow in circulation and the glands. Its colour is rich brown. The vibration is very calming emotionally.

**Nutrition**

Avoid sugar, salt (directly affects blood pressure, leads to hypertension), preserved and processed food. Use plenty of olive oil which is stable and beneficial. Make sure that other cold-pressed oils you use are fresh and stored out of the sun, and avoid processed oils, margarine and shortening. Cut down on fried food, animal fats, butter, cream and dairy fats.

Eat plenty of alkaline vegetables, sprouts and fruit. Complex carbohydrates - whole grains, pulses and seeds are beneficial, particularly oats. Oily fish, like mackerel and salmon, can reduce the tendency to blood clotting and lower blood pressure.

**Supplements**

Have a full maintenance programme, adding vitamins B6, (100-300mg), plus B complex, C complex (3500mg including bioflavonoids) E (starting below 200iu and cautiously raising level over several months to 1000iu) which will lower dangerous LDL cholesterol, strengthen the internal linings and the tissues of the circulatory system, and reduce plaque, clotting and hypertension.

To protect from damage from oxidation - for example

if you have atherosclerosis, or have had years of poor diet, especially the wrong fats and oils, if you've been a smoker or been exposed to pollution - the classic supplements are the 'ACES', vitamin A as beta carotene (25,000 iu), vitamins C and E, as above, and selenium (50 mcg).

A full strength multimineral supplement should contain enough calcium and magnesium to maintain the heart. Iron, potassium, zinc, copper and chromium are also needed. Germanium in safe organic form has been found to benefit circulation.

EPA derived from fish oil and GLA from evening primrose and other sources have both been found to help to inhibit clotting and keep the blood flowing freely.

## Other Aids

Learning to relax as well as exercise with full, deep breathing is very important. Visualise the whole system, and particularly imbalanced organs working harmoniously. Start with the lungs, and imagine blood being refreshed and renewed here, before going back to the heart and from here to the whole body through the arteries. Imagine the arteries clear and healthy. Imagine blood being continuously filtered and actively purified by the kidneys. Imagine all tissues of the body being bathed in healthy oxygenated blood, and the blood returning through the veins to the heart. Imagine that all the right nutrients enter the blood as it goes through the digestive organs. Feel that healing and balance come to you with each breath.

*References:*
1. *I. Adamu, P. Joseph, K. Augusti. Experientia 38. 1982.*
   *O. Sodimi, Joseph, Augusti. Experientia 40. 1984.*
2. *A. Quereshi et al. Lipids 18. 1983.*
3. *R. Passwater. Supernutrition for Healthy Hearts. Thorsons. 977.*
4. *Editorial. The Lancet. 28 May 1983.*
5. *J.M. Lundberg, A. Saria. Nature 302:251-3. 1983.*
6. *M.T. Murray. The 21st Century Herbal. Vita-Line.*

# Herbal C    *Colds and Congestion*

As well as for health promotion, useful in these conditions:

Asthma, bronchitis, common cold, coughs, hayfever, lung congestion, rhinitis, sinusitis, sore throat.
*(For any serious or lasting condition consult your practitioner)*

| | | |
|---|---|---|
| **Boneset** | herb | *Eupatorium perfoliatum* |
| **Catnip** | herb | *Nepeta cataria* |
| **Horehound** | herb | *Marrubium vulgare* |
| **Lemon verbena** | herb | *Lippia citriodora* |
| **Mint** | herb | *Mentha piperita* |
| **Sage** | herb | *Salvia officinalis* |
| **Yarrow** | herb | *Achillea millefolium* |

As powder up to 1/3 gram of each herb daily, or 40mgs of each per tablet, 2-8 daily. Courses of no longer than four months.

## The Body

Most people are only too familiar with cold symptoms - nose and sinus filled with mucus, eyes and head heavy, sore throat, congested lungs, coughs, sniffs, aches and fevers.

The body usually eliminates waste products and toxins by converting them in liver, blood and lymph and excreting them through the kidneys, gall, colon, sweat glands and mucus membranes.

Mucus membrane

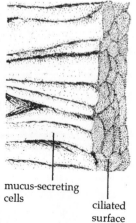

mucus-secreting cells

ciliated surface

Respiratory organs

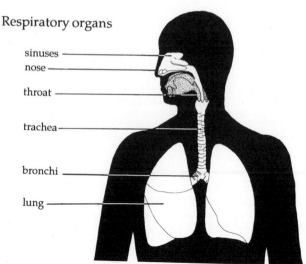

sinuses

nose

throat

trachea

bronchi

lung

A cold is the overloading of one elimination channel, the mucus membranes of nose, throat , lungs, and points to the likelihood of congestion in other channels. Toxic mucus invites bacteria to breed, producing more irritating material. The whole system warms up, speeds its metabolism to increase the conversion and elimination of toxins. When the delicate membranes have been sensitised, any irritation or allergic reaction to food and/or dust and pollen will set off similar symptoms.

Nearly every intestine which has been subject to a normally poor diet makes copious amounts of mucus because of toxicity, putrefaction and irritation. Irritation and mucus production becomes a whole-body problem. Mucus is released directly in lungs and nose, especially when urine and sweat cannot cope with the level. So prevention of cold and hayfever-like symptoms must involve cleansing as well as soothing.

## The Combination

Lemon verbena and boneset gently clear the intestines, yarrow, catnip and boneset cleanse the blood and the liver. yarrow and catnip stimulate perspiration, increasing skin elimination, stimulate the lymphatic system and tone the blood. With sage and lemon verbena they aid glandular control to calm fever.

Boneset and horehound break and clear phlegm and catarrh. mint, horehound and catnip together soothe coughs. Mint and sage are antiseptic cleansers and alleviate sore throat.

Mint and lemon verbena allow relaxation and sleep.

## The Herbs
*Boneset*

Boneset was a favourite remedy of the North American Indians who called it "ague weed", but it got its name from "break-bone fever", a particularly painful flu which it treated successfully. It has been used for the fever of malaria and typhoid as well as flu [1].

Boneset acts slowly and persistently stimulating the defences of the body, particularly the protective white cells, while keeping fever under control. It is a noted cleanser stimulating the stomach and liver to greater efficiency and increasing bile production. It helps restore elimination in the skin, encouraging perspiration, and in the colon, where it clears excessive mucus and putrefying material.

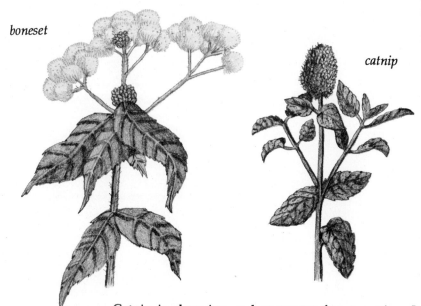

boneset

catnip

**Catnip**

Catnip is cleansing and promotes free sweating. It maintains activity in the blood and lymph and mildly stimulates the glands.It is known as one of the best and most gentle nervines. The tea has been used in the South Apalachians in the U.S. as a specific cold remedy since the 18th century.

**Horehound**

Horehound is the great mucus clearer, working throughout the body to break down hardened mucus and expel it from the colon, lungs and lymph ducts and nodes. It is mildly diuretic. It is noted for all lung troubles and coughs, Culpepper reports that "it helpeth to expectorate tough phlegm from the chest", and Gerrard says, "a most singular remedy against the cough and wheezing of the lungs". [2].

**Lemon verbena**

Lemon verbena's soothing oils work mainly on the autonomic nerve control of muscles. So it is particularly useful to improve digestion and relaxation of the whole body. But also it will work on the bronchi and the lungs to ease coughing and inflammation and promote cleansing.

**Mint**

Mint's oils are delightful to smell and immediately start to clear the nose and sinuses. In attacks of hayfever, mint was one of the few smells which used to calm my red and inflamed nose and eyes. It is a good digestive aid and prevents nausea

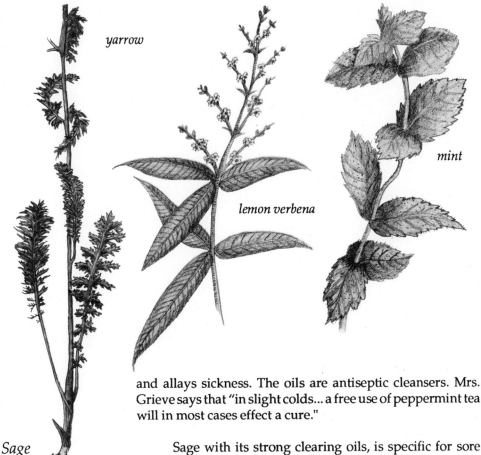

*yarrow*

*mint*

*lemon verbena*

and allays sickness. The oils are antiseptic cleansers. Mrs. Grieve says that "in slight colds... a free use of peppermint tea will in most cases effect a cure."

*Sage*              Sage with its strong clearing oils, is specific for sore throats, inflamed tonsils and heavy heads. Gerrard says, "a most singular remedy against the couch and wheezing of the lungs", and Mrs. Grieve reports that, "In Sussex... to munch sage leaves on nine consecutive mornings, whilst fasting, was a country cure for ague" (3). It stimulates digestion and cleanses the blood, and its effect on the whole body, particularly its ability to dispel depression, is so powerful that the Romans named it the "salvation" herb.

*Yarrow*            Yarrow, while promoting perspiration, prevents excess watery secretions in the rest of the body, and is recommended for severe colds and the start of fevers. The dry powdered leaves were used throughout Europe as a snuff to cleanse the head and sinuses of mucus. Yarrow also calms soreness and helps to heal damaged tissues.

73

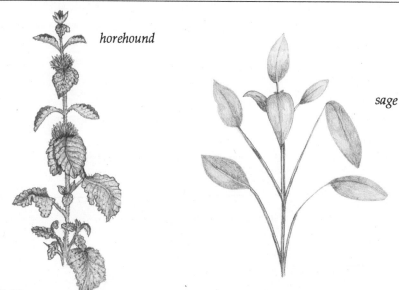

*horehound*

*sage*

**The Mixture**

The mixture smells light, airy and clearing, with a bitter-smooth background taste, and breathing it alone has a strong effect on the nose lungs and sinuses. The leaves of the plants convert sunlight to unique warming oils, but they mostly enjoy damp airy conditions which lends them strength in working with the elements of air and water.

**Nutrition**

Clear the digestive system of mucus by fasting on highly fibrous, non-mucus-producing raw fruits and vegetables. Dairy produce, wheat products, particularly when refined, meat and all processed food is likely to stimulate mucus production. For acute colds and inflammation fast on fruit juice, vegetable juice and water. Don't feed a cold - you are simply overloading the system and providing more food for bacteria. Germs particularly love excess sugar! Cut down salt too, because it often makes up a large part of the mucus you are trying to get rid of, and it irritates sensitive membranes.

Allergic reactions are often caused by insufficient digestion, and it is most important to clear this area to prevent hayfever and asthma.

**Supplements**

In addition to a maintenance level of vitamins and minerals:
Vitamin C (for prevention 1-3 grams; during severe
symptoms 10-20 grams daily).

Vitamin A, the membrane healer (normally 25,000iu), during symptoms up to 200,000iu daily for one week.

B3 (100mg) with B complex (75mg of each of the main B vitamins).

Zinc (50mg chelated or faster action by chewing zinc lozenges).

Digestive enzymes to aid complete digestion and internal cleansing.

Herbal D to cleanse. Herbal I in flu and fever.

**Other Aids**

Cold symptoms are quite stressful, and stress increases allergic reactions like hayfever and asthma. So stress reduction, regular exercise and support for the adrenals, and the whole glandular system will help. This will relieve pressure on the immune system, which is at the 'front line of defence' against cold viruses.

Visualise the body clearing of mucus and calming irritated membranes. See the whole body being soothed and cleared.

Recognise that the cleansing process is leaving you more healthy. Examine how your symptoms affect you emotionally and mentally. Very often we escape by getting ill. Maybe next time you can escape before you get a cold. Use exercise or sauna to keep temperatures high and sweat the cold out. Wrap yourself up and stay warm during fevers. Many viruses and bacteria are less virulent at slightly elevated temperatures.

*References:*
1. B. Griggs. Green Pharmacy. Jill Norman and Hobhouse. 1981.
2. Mrs. M. Grieve. A Modern Herbal. Penguin. 1977.
3. Ibid.

# Herbal D  *Detoxify and Cleanse*

As well as for health promotion, useful in these conditions:

Aches, acne, backache (kidneys), boils, chronic constipation, cystitus, drug toxins, eczema, energy low, hepatitis, infections, jaundice, kidney congestion, liver congestion, psoriasis, poisoning (gases, heavy metals, drugs, insecticides, fertilisers, nicotine, preservatives, food additives, all pollutants), rashes, sluggishness, sores, swollen lymph glands.
*(For any serious or lasting condition consult your practitioner)*

| | | |
|---|---|---|
| **Burdock** | root | *Arctium lappa* |
| **Dandelion** | root | *Taraxacum officinale* |
| **Sarsaparilla** | root | *Smilax officinale* |
| **Yellow dock** | root | *Rumex crispus* |

80mg of each as powder or per tablet, 2-8 daily. Courses of no longer than 3 months.

**The Body**

In natural healing, perhaps the most important organ to notice is the colon, or large intestine. Being at the end of the digestive process it gets to deal with the end results of all the material we swallow. Its chief function is to withdraw fluid from the waste material into the body. Along with this the end-results of bacterial action are absorbed. Bacteria convert a proportion of cellulose into sugars, produce some B vitamins and perform many other useful functions for us, but they will only do this if we encourage the right ones by eating the right foods. There is considerable opportunity to exchange toxins and nutrients through the colon wall, and this organ can be considered eliminative and absorptive.

Eating poisons such as preservatives, salt and additives, eating excessive meat, fat, overcooked and badly combined foods will destroy the beneficial bacteria and encourage poison-producing bacteria. The putrefaction irritates the colon which produces mucus. Over the long term the mucus solidifies to produce a thick covering to the colon tissue, a constant source of poisons and a barrier to correct cleansing.

The liver receives the blood direct from the digestive system and its work is to modify blood chemistry. Foods are inter-converted, stored and released, poisons and toxins are destroyed, neutralised or diluted and, as far as possible, the correct balance is maintained. However, the liver may be overloaded by toxins from food, from the environment, from infection or from internal imbalance. Toxic internal imbalances arise due to excesses of certain foods, like sugar, or deficiencies of other molecules like vitamins and minerals. Products of intermediate metabolism can overwhelm the tissues, come into the blood and arrive at the liver. We may also be trying to deal with heavy metal toxins, like lead, chemicals like DDT and drugs like antibiotics or artificial hormones.

When the liver is unable to detoxify, the job is taken up by the lymphatic system and its roving white cells. They will surround, and try to digest and engulf poisons. But if they are overwhelmed by internal toxicity, less protection is available against infection and malignancy.

Cross-section of the colon

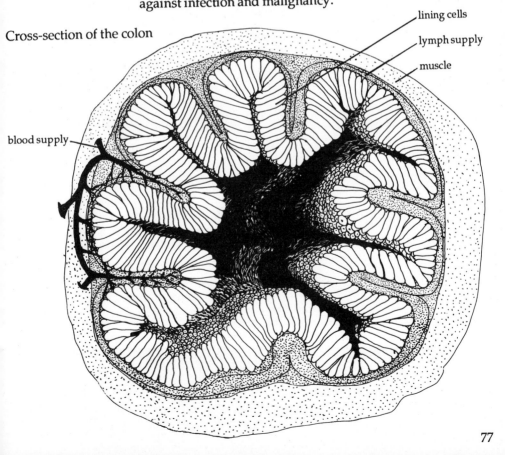

lining cells

lymph supply

muscle

blood supply

77

Eliminative Organs

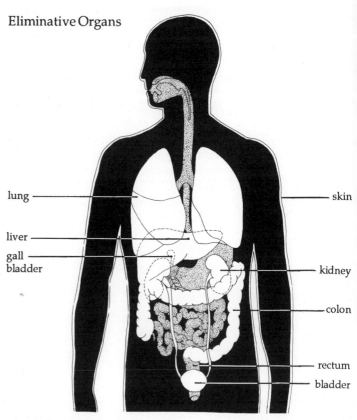

lung — skin

liver —

gall bladder — — kidney

— colon

— rectum

— bladder

Finally toxins will try to exit through the main channels of elimination, firstly through the kidneys and urinary system. Assuming the colon cannot be used to excrete because it is already too dirty, the skin may be involved, giving body odour, acne and rashes, or greasy skin. Or we may use the mucus membranes of the nose and throat, developing a cold. Wherever toxins emerge they may attract bacteria or viruses to breed on them. So when certain toxins are produced in the lungs we may be heading for pneumonia or other infections.

*Detoxification therefore is basic to any natural return to balance and health.*

## The Combination

Burdock and yellow dock are mildly laxative and cleanse the digestive system, gradually loosening old deposits from the colon wall. With dandelion and sarsaparilla they detoxify the liver promoting bile, and neutralise some poisons directly. All are powerful blood cleansers.

Sarsaparilla and burdock stimulate sweating and clear the skin. Burdock and yellow dock work through the lymphatic system to the skin, encouraging the effectiveness of white cells. Dandelion and burdock clean the kidneys.

### The Herbs
*Burdock*

Burdock, containing sulphur, iron and B vitamins, is attuned to aiding protein metabolism in skin, lymph and blood. So it reduces toxic internal imbalance. It neutralises and eliminates poisons and stimulates the liver and kidneys. It helps the colon throw off sticky mucus, at the same time reducing inflammation. Jethro Kloss [1] mentions burdock for "scrofula, canker sores, syphilis, gonorrhoea and leprosy"

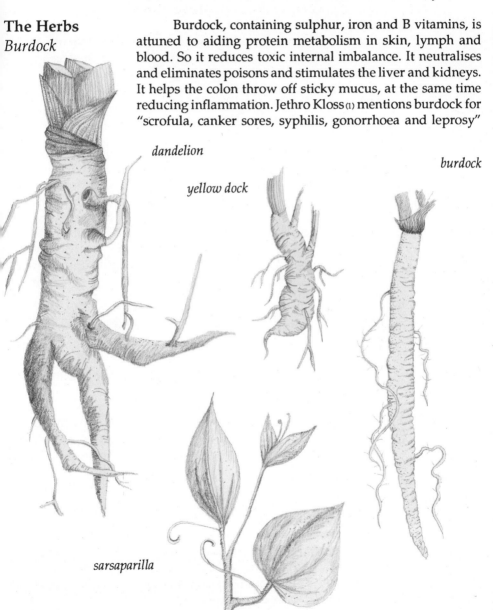

*dandelion*

*yellow dock*

*burdock*

*sarsaparilla*

79

and Priest and Priest [2] say that it removes accumulated waste from skin and mucus membranes and "is specific for eruptions on the head, face and neck, and for acute irritable and inflammatory conditions", such as "eczema, psoriasis, dermatitis - boils, carbuncles, styes and sores."

## Dandelion

Dandelion is known as a powerful cure for intractable liver congestion, increasing the flow of bile which helps release toxins and is slightly laxative. It is very high in minerals and is a blood builder. High potassium content makes it an excellent balance for excessive sodium from salt, and dandelion helps to clear and balance the kidneys.

## Sarsaparilla

Sarsaparilla is a common spring tonic, it helps balance male and female hormones and aids associated skin problems, being an excellent acne remedy. Nelson [3] reports that it was used to relieve syphilitic sores and for a variety of skin ailments. It has been shown to be effective in treating psoriasis - in one controlled study 62% of psoriasis patients improved and 18% had complete clearing of the skin [4]. It mainly seems to act by binding bacterial toxins that enter through the colon into the bloodstream [5]. It is very soothing and reduces excessive mucus.

## Yellow dock

Yellow dock works strongly on glandular swellings, swollen lymph glands and has even been used to help limit cancers. It encourages old mucus deposits to swell and strip off from the colon wall. It has a history of use in treating skin eruptions and urticaria (nettle rash).

## The Mixture

The mixture is strongly aromatic with a mixture of bitter cleansers and volatile warm oils. It is brown-red, strong and rooty, reaching deep through the body with the feeling of fire and earth.

## Nutrition

Eat raw fibrous vegetables, sprouted seeds, beans, lentils etc.,and fruit. (80% of diet). Have best quality whole foods in addition - yoghurt, low salt cheeses, fish, eggs, organic meat, mixed grains and pulses. Cold pressed (un-processed) oils, but no fried food. Cooked potatoes in jackets, bananas, little or no wheat products. No salt. No sugar, but honey, molasses and fruit sugar in moderation.

No processed, canned, frozen or reconstituted food of

any kind. Psyllium husks are an excellent way of drawing encrusted mucus out of the colon (1 tsp. in water 3 times daily). See also the colon cleansing programme (6). Drink 4 glasses of springwater daily. An occasional fast on vegetables only, or fruit only for a few days helps to speed cleansing.

## Supplements

In addition to a maintenance programme the following supplements my be useful: vitamin C is the great detoxifying vitamin 2-10 grams daily. B complex (75mg major B's) is needed for all metabolic processes involved in detoxifying, together with other vitamins and minerals. For lead use vitamin C as calcium ascorbate amino acid chelate (1-3 grams) and zinc 50mg. B3, niacin (100mg) often causes a beneficial skin flush which can help clear toxicity from the whole skin area. Chlorella - an ancient microscopic alga - also has unique detoxifying properties. 25- 30 tablets or 6 grams per day are suggested for optimal detoxification. These should be taken on an empty stomach, taken all at once or in divided doses.

## Other Aids

Saunas and sweat-promoting exercise are most important to aid detoxification. Use of water in Turkish baths, salt water bathing, Epsom salts baths, or fresh water are also excellent.

Avoid using deodorants based on aluminium since they are toxic and tend to prevent elimination of other toxins. Internal cleansing is the way to deodorise! Enemas with pure water, diluted wheat grass juice or weak coffee are an excellent way to clear the loose material from the colon and stimulate cleansing.

Daily, imagine your colon, liver, lymph, blood, kidneys, lungs and skin changing from their overloaded and dirty state to pure bright cleanliness and health.

*References:*
1. *J. Kloss. Back to Eden. Lifeline Books. 1972.*
2. *Priest A.W. and Priest L.R. Herbal Medication. L.N. Fowler. 1982.*
3. *A. Nelson. Medical Botany. E. & S. Livingstone. 1951.*
4. *F.M. Thurman. New Eng. J. Med. 227:128-33. 1942.*
5. *M. Murray. The 21st Century Herbal. Vita Line.*
6. *B. Wright. Cleansing the Colon. Green Press. 1987.*

# Herbal E    *Eye Tonic*

As well as for health promotion, useful in these conditions:

Blepharitis, cataract, conjunctivitis, corneal irritation, dimming of sight, hayfever, infections of the eye, long and short sightedness, styes, watery eyes.
*(For any serious or lasting condition consult your practitioner.)*

| **Eyebright** | herb | *Euphrasia officinalis* |
| **Golden seal** | herb | *Hydrastis canadensis* |
| **Rosemary** | herb | *Rosmarinus officinalis* |
| **Rue** | herb | *Ruta graveolens* |

78mgs of each except golden seal 50mgs as powder or per tablet, 2-5 daily. Courses of no longer than 3 months.

*This combination should not be used during pregnancy as rue is a uterine stimulant at high dosage.Golden seal reduces B vitamin synthesis in the colon, so supplement with B complex and have several months' break after each course.*

**The Body**

Perhaps our most-used organ of perception the eyes are especially vulnerable to the world beyond the body.

The membranes, and their lubricating fluid from the tear ducts, are subject to air pollution and irritation daily. They must be maintained by making sure that the tear fluid itself is clean and that no wastes are produced allowing infection to be set up.

Internally the eyes reflect the health of the whole body. The muscles used to adjust the lens and direct the eye must retain their flexibility by being assured of supplies of oxygen and nutrients and no toxins. The cornea, lens and internal fluid are dependant on the blood supplying these critical factors too. Also the blood vessels must be maintained to prevent haemorrhage from clouding sight. The nerve supply and the receptive cells of the retina are obviously essential to maintain at optimum health. These highly sensitive nerve cells are maintained in balance between the needs of our whole organism - physical, emotional, mental and spiritual - particularly between attention and relaxation. An eye tonic must be able to stimulate the clearing of deposits and if possible pursuade the body to eliminate elsewhere. It must also encourage the particular tissues to absorb the nutrients needed for health, and maintain a consistent energy and flexibility of response.

## The Eye

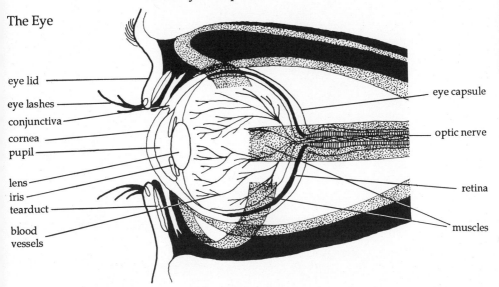

eye lid
eye lashes
conjunctiva
cornea
pupil

lens
iris
tearduct

blood
vessels

eye capsule

optic nerve

retina

muscles

## The Combination

Eyebright and golden seal help eliminate membrane conditions like conjunctivitis by cleansing, cooling and disinfecting the membranes.

With rosemary they are powerful remedies for allergies and hayfever. Golden seal and rosemary are antiseptic, and can be used externally for this purpose.

Eyebright and rue are specific for muscle tone, stimulating the digestive system, liver and kidneys, circulation and nervous system, providing a background of clean efficiency which may take the toxic load off the eyes.

## The Herbs
### *Eyebright*

Eyebright as the name indicates has long been used as a cure-all for eyes, effective in infections, weakness, opthalmia and cataracts. Culpepper said "if the herb was as much used as it is neglected, it would half spoil the spectacle makers trade" [1]. It is astringent, drying up discharges, and useful in all allergic reactions and 'red-eye' conditions as it calms, cools and soothes the conjunctival membranes [2].

### *Golden Seal*

Golden seal, a catalyst of the other herbs, is traditionally used with Eyebright. It stimulates the immune system

83

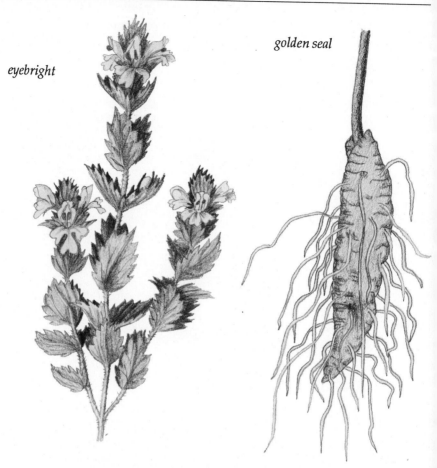

eyebright

golden seal

to clear viral, bacterial and fungal infections. It is a strong antiseptic cleanser, and the top healer of mucus membranes, and the conjunctiva. American Indians used it as their main eye medicine.

**Rosemary**

Rosemary, with its aromatic oil is a nervine and disinfectant, soothing allergic reactions and toning the whole body. Rosemary will also be working in the background to stimulate the digestive process, particularly the liver, and so help to remove toxic and allergenic particles from the body.

**Rue**

Rue is nervine, soothing the nerves involved in vision, and well known as a nightmare cure. It is known that dreams affect the visual pathways, so rue benefits the brain-eye connection and maintains resilience in nerve tissue. Rue

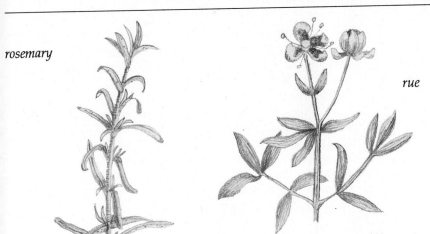

*rosemary*

*rue*

increases blood flow to smooth muscle, and is therefore beneficial to lens and pupil, as well as to the digestive system. It should not be used during pregnancy, however, as it also stimulates the muscles of the uterus.

**The Mixture**

With the strong aromatic oils of rue and rosemary and the bitterness of golden seal, the powdered herbs affect eyes and sinuses directly. The yellow-green colour reflects clearing water, restoring earth and refreshing air elements.

*An Example*

A remarkable illustration of some effects of the combination is given in this letter received from Mrs. Carr:

*"My sister, who is very short sighted, complained of achey and itchy eyes. She looked very uncomfortable and the doctor's anti-biotics had not improved anything. She took these 4 tablets of the combination three times a day] and found a rapid improvement. BUT she wears soft lenses and those became a beautiful shade of pink. [After a month she felt better and stopped taking the herbs]. She decided to carry on wearing the lenses and little by little they returned to their original colour. It is an odd thing, but does not at all diminish the great efficacy of the eyebright tablets."*

Unfortunately we could not test the pink substance taken up by the lenses, but it seems quite likely that this was a toxic colouring released as a result of using the herbs.

**Nutrition**

Food for the eyes has traditionally included all the vitamin A foods like carrots and liver. In fact all red and yellow vegetables and a number of green ones, like spinach and parsley, are high in beta carotene which is converted to vitamin A in the body according to need.

All kinds of degenerative eye diseases can be avoided by replacing processed, "chemicalised", and salted and sugared food and drink with real, fresh and mainly raw food. The cleansing diet in the Herbal Detox section is suitable for all eye conditions.

After the diet is free of toxic additives, it may be profitable to find out if there are allergic reactions to any foods or drinks which affect sensitive tissues like the eye membranes. You can do this by starting with a fast and introducing foods one by one. You should eliminate any you have a reaction to for a few months while you work on improving your digestion and overall health.

## Supplements

Vitamin A, retinol, is used directly in the retina where it allows production of visual pigment used when there are fast changes in light, or when detail or night vision is important. A is also needed to restore health of all the eye membranes (during healing 25,000-100,000 iu daily). To be safe, the greatest proportion of this should be taken as beta carotene. Amongst other nutrients vitamin C and zinc are perhaps the most important. B2 (100-300mg) is specific for itchy red eyes and all acidic skin inflammations. These should be added to the maintenance programme.

## Other Aids

A weak tea can be made of the combination (one tablet to a pint) and when it has settled, cooled and been strained the eyes may be bathed three times a day.

Chronic conditions often need a whole-body approach which can undo long-lasting imbalances, so it is important not to consider the eyes in isolation. Visualising is an activity which itself will exercise the visual pathways. When the eye is imagined as a complex organ of different tissues and you visualise the cleansing, balancing and support of each of the tissues, its health is enormously enhanced. Recommended for the improvement of the muscles and lens: The Bates Method [3]. The way you see things describes your feelings and thought as well as your sight. Cultivate your openness to seeing everything, your curiosity and attention to detail.

*References:*
1. *Mrs. Grieve. op. cit.*
2. *Priest and Priest. op. cit.*
3. *Information from the Secretary,49 Queen Anne St. London W1.*

# Herbal F   *Female Tonic*

As well as for health promotion, useful in these conditions:

Afterpains, amenorrhoea, breast conditions, childbirth (relaxation in, membrane condition, recovery from etc.), glandular imbalance, infertility, menstruation (irregularity, pain, blood loss etc.), ovaries (cysts, abnormalities) pregnancy, uterine conditions, vaginitis and infections.
*(During pregnancy or for any lasting or serious condition, consult your practitioner.)*

| | | |
|---|---|---|
| **Liquorice** | root | *Glycyrrhiza glabra* |
| **Mistletoe** | herb | *Viscum alba* |
| **Black Cohosh** | root | *Cimicifuga racemosa* |
| **Raspberry** | leaf | *Rubus idaeus* |

75mg of each as powder or per tablet, 2-6 daily. Courses of no longer than 4 months.

## The Body

The mature female body works in cycles of menstruation which change normally as a result of pregnancy and over a period known as menopause.

The cycles, the development of the feminine body shape and characteristics, pregnancy, menopause and the condition of sexual organs, breasts and much of the female biochemistry are all under the influence of the glandular system. The system uses the ovaries, adrenal glands and pituitary gland as the sources of hormones which balance each other through feedback systems. The brain has access to the pituitary gland via the hypothalamus, so that thought affects and is affected by hormonal balance.

Four major types of premenstrual tension syndrome (PMTS) have been described [1]. PMT-A is premenstrual anxiety, irritability and nervous tension. PMT-H goes with water and salt retention, bloating, breast pain and weight gain. PMT-C is associated with craving and eating sugary food, followed by palpitations, fatigue, headaches and shakiness. PMT-D means depression, insomnia, confusion and suicidal feelings. There are particular recommendations for each of these types.

Besides helping to balance the hormones, a natural

87

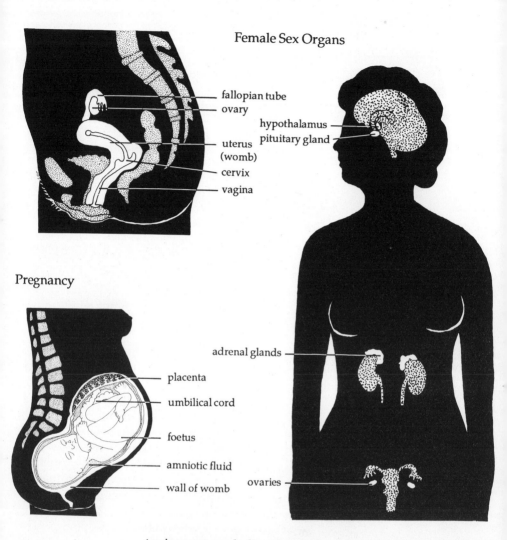

Female Sex Organs

fallopian tube
ovary
hypothalamus
pituitary gland
uterus
(womb)
cervix
vagina

Pregnancy

adrenal glands

placenta

umbilical cord

foetus

amniotic fluid

wall of womb    ovaries

tonic must work directly on the organs involved. The fallopian tubes, uterus and vagina have sensitive membranes, which particularly in the case of the uterus, build up, secrete and are replaced in the course of the menstrual cycle. In pregnancy they go through further changes. The placenta is built up with secretory cells and a very full circulatory exchange which monitors blood supply to the embryo. Muscular relaxation, promotion of blood and lymph supply, cleaning and disinfecting and nuturing properties are needed in the herbs we use.

**The Combination**
Liquorice and black cohosh contain natural hormones which help mediate menstruation, comfortable menopause, uterine and sexual development.

Mistletoe and raspberry leaf help normalise menstruation, preventing pain and excess bleeding.

Liquorice and raspberry leaf are strengthening and cleansing for the membranes of the sexual organs, uterus and fallopian tubes.

**The Herbs**
*Black cohosh*
Black cohosh was used by American Indians for all female complaints. It is a source of natural oestrogen and other substances which aid the balance of sex hormones. It also prevents muscle spasm and cramps, and promotes relaxation in childbirth, hence its American Indian name of 'squawroot'.

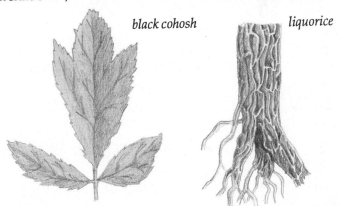

*black cohosh*          *liquorice*

*Liquorice*
Liquorice is a powerful clearer of mucus congestion, and aids kidney, bladder and vaginal ailments. It is a blood purifier and a mild laxative. Its hormonal activities make it a tonic for the adrenal glands, in increasing the anti-inflammatory effect of the hormone cortisol (2) and thereby reducing discomfort in PMTS, in their role in maintaining mineral levels in blood and bone, and in helping to normalise the production of sex hormones. Liquorice also has valuable soothing properties, is recommended for catarrh of the urinary tract and helps prevent thrush and vaginal infections. In high concentration it can cause problems for people with high blood pressure.

*Mistletoe*
Mistletoe, containing calcium, magnesium, sodium and potassium, is a strong nervine and antispasmodic and its gentle anaesthetic properties make it useful for menstrual or

pregnancy pains. It stimulates the kidneys, reducing blood pressure and increasing urine. It checks excessive menstruation. It has been found to inhibit malignant growths, and in druidic lore was the great protector, always allied to the female energy.

*Raspberry*

Raspberry leaf, a traditional pregnancy herb, eliminates morning sickness, strengthens the uterus, prevents the pains of childbirth and after-birth pain and helps prevent birth defects. As it contains and aids assimilation of vitamins A,B,C,E and minerals calcium, magnesium, phosphorus, potassium and sulphur it is important in the regulation of the glandular system, membrane surfaces and the placenta. It is also recommended for thrush, irregular periods and as a mild laxative.

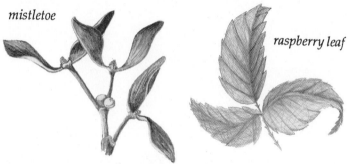

*mistletoe*

*raspberry leaf*

**The Mixture**

The mixture is light brown-green and combines earthy roots with very fibrous, airy leaves of raspberry, and the tougher watery stems and leaves of mistletoe. These herbs have long traditions of working with the deep natural forces in a quiet rhythmic way.

**Nutrition**

An alkaline diet is best for glandular balance. Some foods which stress the glands and should be avoided are sugar, salt, excessive coffee and alcohol, preserved and processed foods. PMT-A sufferers should avoid dairy products, especially before a period. All types are sensitive to sugar and salt. PMT-D should be especially careful to avoid toxic additives and have a balanced diet.

For vaginal and other infections, a detoxifying diet, as recommended with Herbal Detox is essential.

Pregnancy obviously requires the best possible diet with gradually increasing amounts of protein and mineral-high foods.

**Supplements**

For all PMT conditions, in addition to a maintenance programme, B6 100-500 mg and magnesium 200-400 mg are recommended. Evening primrose and other oils containing GLA are also effective.

Vitamin C 1-4 g extra, E 1000 iu (except where there are heart or high blood pressure problems), RNA/DNA 500mg or female gland extracts (2-4 tablets.) are also used in cases where a rebalancing of the whole glandular system needs to take place. Where there are stress-related problems, vitamin B5 (500-1000mg) more C and ginseng may be useful.

Menopausal symptoms, infertility, menstrual irregularity and mastitis are among the imbalances that respond well to vitamin E and supplemental boron particularly. To prevent osteoporosis and the mineral imbalances which many women suffer after menopause, take extra magnesium and calcium, together with boron 3 mg a part of your supplement programme.

In pregnancy supplementation should be very adequate in all vitamins and minerals, at the top end of the maintenance level. A balanced amino acid complex would also ensure adequate supplies of the protein building blocks needed for making tissues, enzymes and all essential body chemicals.

**Other Aids**

Female hormones are used as contraceptives and to treat symptoms of menopause through hormone replacement therapy. In both cases there is the possibility of severe side effects of daily exposure. Although not as direct or guaranteed, the natural methods are certainly safer.

The brain connects all through to the hypothalamus and hence pituitary gland. This means that our thoughts and basic ideas and beliefs directly affect our hormones. If you want to improve or change anything in this area, forming mental pictures works directly. Develop relaxation, centred breathing and confidence. Surround yourself with images of the positive state you want to reach. This is also a way of making a powerful link to a growing child in the uterus. The child will respond to herbs, nutrition, emotions and thoughts and all kinds of influences from its environment.

*References:*
1. G.S. Goei, J.L. Ralston, G.E. Abraham. J. Appl. Nutr. 34:4. 1982.
2. M. Murray. The 21st Century Herbal. Vita Line..

# Herbal G  *Gastro-Intestinal Tonic*

As well as for health promotion, useful in these conditions:

Appendicitis, catarrh, colic, colitis, constipation, diarrhoea, diverticulosis, flatulence (gas), gastro-enteritis, nausea, nervous stomach, piles, ulcers (stomach, duodenum, colon).
*(For any serious or lasting condition consult your practitioner.)*

| | | |
|---|---|---|
| **Cayenne** | fruit | *Capsicum minimum* |
| **Comfrey** | herb | *Symphytum officinale* |
| **Golden seal** | root | *Hydrastis canadensis* |
| **Slippery elm** | bark | *Ulmus fulva* |

As powder or per tablet 85mg cayenne, comfrey, 65mg golden seal, 100mg slippery elm. 2-6 daily. Courses of no longer than 4 months. Golden seal reduces B vitamin synthesis in the colon, so supplement with B complex and have several months' break between courses.

**The Body**

To see the digestive system more easily let us follow the progress of a meal. Mixed with saliva, each mouthful progresses down the muscular oesophagus through a valve and into the stomach. The stomach is lined with protective mucus membrane with secretory cells producing hydrochloric acid, pepsin, and other protein and fat-digesting enzymes. The stomach wall is quite muscular, has connective tissue

Cross section of the small intestine

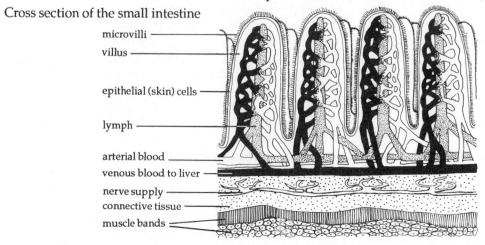

microvilli
villus
epithelial (skin) cells
lymph
arterial blood
venous blood to liver
nerve supply
connective tissue
muscle bands

linings and a good blood and nerve supply. If the wall is ulcerated through stress and inadequate nutrition, the acid needed for digestion becomes irritating.

After 1-3 hours our meal passes out of the stomach and into the duodenum where it mixes with alkali and enzymes from the pancreas, and bile for fat dispersal from the gall bladder.

The duodenum is the beginning of more serious absorption which continues in the small intestine, along with production of more enzymes and lubricating juices. The lining becomes more and more frond-like, making a vast surface area very adequately supplied with blood and lymph vessels.

The Gastro-Intestinal System

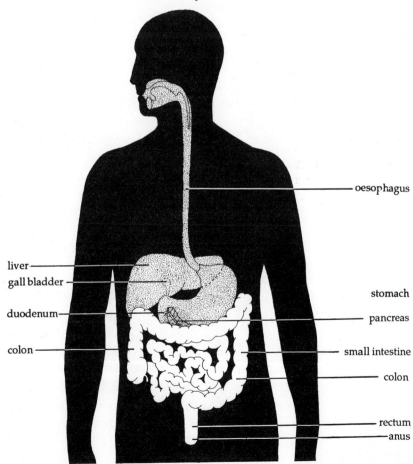

liver

gall bladder

duodenum

colon

oesophagus

stomach

pancreas

small intestine

colon

rectum

anus

Correct alkaline/acid balance, avoidance of aluminium and full production of enzymes is necessary to prevent flatulence, inadequate digestion, and irritating putrefaction which leads to diarrhoea or constipation.

Our meal, hopefully with all nutrients extracted, passes through another valve, past the appendix and into the colon. Here bacteria come into their own, completing digestion, or if our colons are not clean, producing putrefaction. Water is absorbed and faeces produced. If the beneficial balance is correct faeces are soft, bulky and comfortable to pass. If there is putrefaction, the faecal matter and mucus hardens and builds up hard plaque inside the colon. This, together with stress and nutritional lacks predisposes the wall of the colon to ulcers, inflammation and diverticulosis.

Cross section
of the
Small Intestine

muscle layers

fronds or "villi"

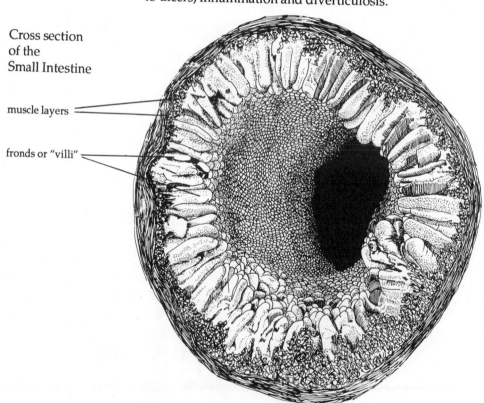

The whole system is coordinated by the nervous system and by messenger hormones. There is a flow of muscular contraction and relaxation which keeps the contents moving.

**The Combination**

Slippery elm and comfrey produce an abundance of mucilage which soothes and cleanses. It helps to dissolve hardened mucus in the colon and clears putrefying material. Cayenne and golden seal are powerful stimulants of mucus and digestive glands, muscles and membranes, keeping nerve and blood supplies active throughout the system.

Slippery elm, comfrey and golden seal work strongly on catarrh and congestion. This is noticed first in the stomach, where the walls are prevented from becoming "soggy" with mucus, and digestion becomes much more efficient.

Golden seal clears and disinfects, allowing cayenne to stimulate and speed healing, while comfrey cleanses and mends and slippery elm nourishes, soothes and carries the mixture while withdrawing mucus.

**The Herbs**
*Cayenne*

Cayenne is a fiery stimulant and it needs to be enclosed in a strong mucilage of the combination. The capsaicin in cayenne abolishes the membrane response to histamine, reducing allergic reactions and the consequent inflammation and mucus production. It selectively stimulates, then blocks nerve fibres in mucus membranes by releasing 'substance P', an unknown biochemical, from nerves [1]. Cayenne is experienced as hot when it comes into contact with the mouth or any skin surface and it stimulates the local blood supply, improving the metabolism of all intestinal tissues and relieving cramps by providing oxygen and nutrients to the underlying muscles. It also heals bleeding and haemorrhoids, clears indigestion and stimulates appetite, increasing enzyme production. It is a good source of vitamins and minerals, notably vitamins A and C, and is a catalyst of other herbs.

*Comfrey*

Comfrey produces an astringent and expectorant mucilage and dries and extracts excess mucus from the intestines. It is a gentle remedy for diarrhoea and dysentery and improves the environment of the colon. The allantoin of comfrey has been demonstrated to speed the repair of connective tissue in skin, bone, gastric and duodenal ulcers. Its use on external skin was reported extensively early this century following the work of Macalister [2]. It was recognised even in the pharmaceutical world - "Allantoin has been used many years by the medical profession to stimulate healthy granulation of tissues" [3] - i.e. cell reproduction and repair.

## Golden Seal

Golden seal, another herbal "amplifier" is a specialist in mucus membranes, clearing catarrh, infection and inflammation. It is mildly laxative, and disinfects, preventing putrefaction, while toning the muscles and stimulating appetite.

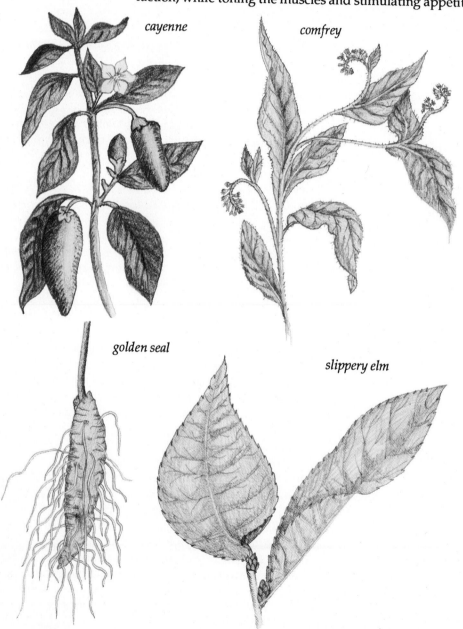

*cayenne*

*comfrey*

*golden seal*

*slippery elm*

*Slippery elm*

Slippery elm is the most widely used gastro-intestinal healer because of its mucilage, which is softening, lubricating, strengthening, healing, nourishing and, above all, soothing. It takes catarrh, toxins and putrefied material with it and provides a healing medium beyond compare.

**The Mixture**

The mixture combines soft pink, green, bright orange and bright yellow, giving a feeling of the strength and softness of the combination. It is fire and earth disolved in the watery element.

**Nutrition**

The gastro-intestinal system gets direct experience of all the rubbish we tend to feed ourselves and suffers most directly from any lack of nutrients.

So here above all we need to base our diet on alkaline intake of fresh vegetables, sprouted seeds and pulses and fruit, organic if possible. Our proteins should be simple - mixed grains and pulses, seeds, fish, eggs, yoghurt, low salt, low fat cheese, organically raised meat. Cold pressed, unprocessed oils rather than animal fat, fried food or refined oil. Wholemeal grains rather than refined flours. Honey and molasses and no sugar or sugar-sweetened food or drink. Juices, water, herb teas rather than tea and coffee. Occasional real ale or good wine rather than spirits. Spices, garlic and herbs rather than salt. No salted, preserved, processed or over cooked food. Fibre is already plentiful in this diet and extra wheat bran is not the best way to improve fibre content because it prevents mineral absorption and can cause flatulence. One of the major problems we hear of is flatulence and poor digestion caused by reaction of aluminium with pancreatic juices. So check your cooking pans, foil and utensils.

**Supplements**

In addition to the maintenance levels of supplements these supplements are recommended to boost the functioning of the tissues:

For health of the mucus membrane lining vitamin A (25-100,000 iu, mainly as beta carotene), and the protein building blocks, amino acids, particularly L-glutamine which is used in natural treatment of ulcers. B complex (75mg major B's) for nerves, muscles and all tissues. C complex (2-4 grams) for blood vessels and connective tissue linings, or an ascorbate (C combined with a mineral) when the digestive system is sensitive to acid. E (400-2000iu) for muscle tone and healing membranes, for instance in diverticulosis. (Caution with any circulatory imbalance). Minerals: calcium, magnesium and zinc. Herbal A and D may be relevant. Digestive enzymes, papaya and pancreatin (pancreas enzymes) will boost digestion immediately, lowering putrefaction, gas and irritation and improving absorption.

**Other Aids**

The gastro-intestinal system is easier to feel directly than most other parts of the body. So we have a good idea of the areas that need attention. Visualising the organs in detail, imagine the tissues improving in balance and assure yourself that what you eat is nourishing and helpful. Blessing food, saying grace, or simply being confident that the food is being used for the best possible purposes relaxes and aids the whole digestive process.

Massage can help the system to relax and can be used along with breathing to bring emotional calm to the system.

*References:*
1. *Editorial. The Lancet. 28 May 1983.*
2. *V. Licata. Comfrey and Chlorophyll. Continental Health Res. 1983.*
3. *R.R. Johnson. J. Am. Pharm. Ass. NS7.11. 1967.*

# Herbal H    *Head and Nerves*

As well as for health promotion, useful in these conditions:

Anxiety, asthma, convulsions, cramp, depression, earache, epilepsy, headache, irritability, migraine, nervousness, neuralgia, neuritis, nightmares, oversensitivity, tension, tinnitis.
*(For any serious or lasting condition consult your practitioner)*

| | | |
|---|---|---|
| **Catnip** | herb | *Nepeta cataria* |
| **Lady's slipper** | root | *Cypripedium pubescens* |
| **Lemon verbena** | herb | *Lippia citriodora* |
| **Sage** | herb | *Salvia officinalis* |
| **Scullcap** | herb | *Scutellaria galericulata* |

60mg of each as powder or per tablet, 2-6 daily. Courses of no lomger than 2 months.

**The Body**    The autonomic nervous system controls blood pressure and flow through different parts of the body, affects muscular contraction, secretion and overall activation. Its centres are in the lower brain, ganglia in the spinal region and in the plexuses, such as the solar plexus.

This system controls many of the unconscious reactions which might result in headaches, tension, shakiness and anxiety. These include disturbances in blood supply - in classical migraine blood vessels constrict during the 'build-up period, and then dilate producing pain, inflammation and often nausea. Other headaches follow the line of main arteries in the head, and muscular tension in the head and neck is a very common cause.

The central nervous system is organised differently with sensory nerves, including pain receptors, coming into the spinal cord and brain and motor nerves, which control voluntary muscles, going in the opposite direction.

The two types of nerves are quite similar in structure individually. They consist of a nerve cell body with branches or "axons" which are covered in a fatty sheath. Axons meet at "synapses" where the electro-chemical nerve impulse changes to a chemical "neurotransmitter" allowing it to jump the gap.

Nutrition of the nerve cell comes mainly via the sheath,

and, having no great storage capacity, nerves must have a good supply of the right nutrients always available. Neuro-transmitters are also very adjustable according to supplies of nutrients and modifying chemicals. Where nerves feel over-stimulated or deadened, the synapse is the first place we need to rebalance.

## Autonomic Nervous System

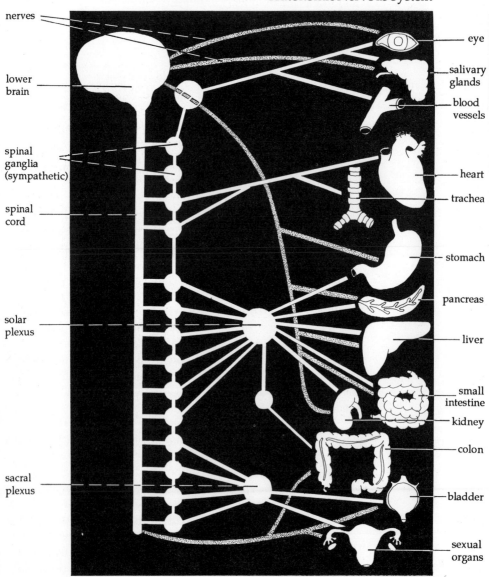

nerves

lower
brain

spinal
ganglia
(sympathetic)

spinal
cord

solar
plexus

sacral
plexus

eye

salivary
glands

blood
vessels

heart

trachea

stomach

pancreas

liver

small
intestine

kidney

colon

bladder

sexual
organs

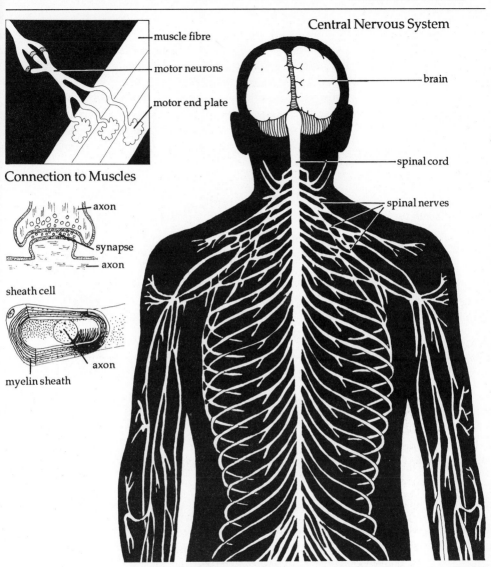

muscle fibre

motor neurons

motor end plate

Central Nervous System

brain

spinal cord

spinal nerves

Connection to Muscles

axon

synapse

axon

sheath cell

axon

myelin sheath

Many poisons, like carbon monoxide gas, lead, DDT and copper, affect nerves and can be cleansed using herbs and nutrients. Stress, involving glands and nerves can rebound on the nervous system increasing allergic reactions, depression and mental tension or illness. Some people have headaches as allergic reaction to substances they have eaten, or breathed in. All the body's functions are monitored by and in turn affect the nerves, so that a natural nerve treatment must work on the whole body.

**The Combination**  Lemon verbena and catnip stimulate and calm the digestive system working on the autonomic nerves' connection to the muscles and digestive glands. Catnip and sage help the blood to throw off toxins. Catnip, lady's slipper, lemon verbena and scullcap are noted muscle relaxants and prevent spasms. The whole combination covers a spectrum of effects directly on the nerves. The oils of the herbs are particularly suited to facilitating the complex feedback systems at nerve synapses.

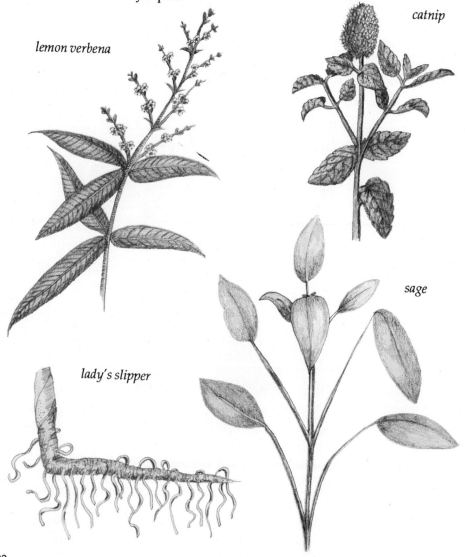

*catnip*

*lemon verbena*

*sage*

*lady's slipper*

**The Herbs**
*Catnip*

Catnip is cleansing and, containing and aiding assimilation of vitamin C, helps detoxify and remove poisons, stimulating the kidneys and sweating. Catnip has a long tradition of use for headaches, hysteria and nightmares. It gives cats ecstasies and may do something similar for human moods too, at least raising depression!

*scullcap*

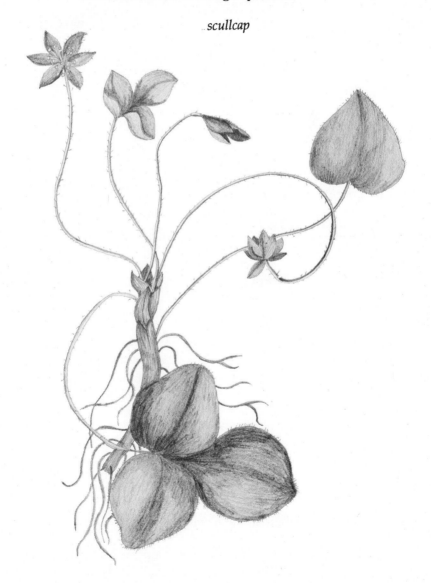

**Lady's slipper**

Lady's slipper, known as "nerve root" is a gentle nerve stimulant and antispasmodic. It aids the transmission of nervous impulses, helping to regulate the autonomic nervous system. It is noted particularly as a muscle relaxant, and is highly recommended for pain and nervous tension resulting from physical conditions [1].

**Lemon verbena**

Lemon verbena, with its soothing oil, aids digestion and relaxes the whole system, working particularly on the autonomic nerve connection to smooth muscle. Since smooth muscle is important in digestion and other "vegetative" or building processes it can be very disrupted during anxiety and over-activation.

**Sage**

Sage is powerfully penetrating and excellent for sinus-associated head pains. It contains vitamin B3 which is used in nerve impulse transmission, has been used successfully to treat schizophrenia in megadoses, and also opens the capillaries. It also contains bioflavonoids which have an anti-allergic effect [2]. Culpepper says sage is "of excellent use to help the memory, warming and quickening of the senses" [3].

**Scullcap**

Scullcap is a traditional cure for hysteria, convulsions, hydrophobia, epilepsy and St. Vitus' Dance. Also a headache and neuralgia herb, it is slightly sedative and stimulates the kidneys. For tension-type imbalances, scullcap is a supreme healer.

## The Mixture

The mixture is strongly aromatic, opening the head and warming the lungs and whole body. It is smooth, leafy and warm, with the elements of air and fire balanced by water.

## Nutrition

The use of sugar, except in natural forms like honey and molasses, strips the nerves of all the nutrients needed to burn it for energy. Salt, as sodium, is used in the nerve impulse itself and taking extra salt in food is not recommended.

Additives and preservatives as well as pollutants affect the nerves directly, so all processed food should be avoided, mineral water or filtered water used, and only real fresh foods eaten.

The best nerve food is fresh vital and high in available nutrients - raw vegetables, sprouts and fruit; fibrous whole grains (soaked or sprouted) wheatgerm, yoghurt and liver (high in B vitamins). Coffee and tea directly affect the nerves, as does chocolate and cocoa. So the balance of these in diet has to be carefully considered. There are sometimes allergies to be considered, and the best way to assess and modify your reactions to food can be found in the Wright Diet (4).

## Supplements

In addition to a maintenance programme, the following supplements may be helpful:

The major nerve vitamin is the B complex (75-100mg major B's). Individual high dose B vitamins are also very effective healers, for instance B3 (100-3000mg), B6 (100-500mg) are used to ground, calm and disolve tension. Choline and inositol (600mg each) are useful natural tranquillisers without side-effects.

Minerals are very important in nerve transmission; (potassium as Herbal K or 100-500mg chelated balances sodium) and the nerve connection to muscles (calcium and magnesium - e.g. dolomite 2-10 tablets), to help relaxation and reduce anxiety. Manganese, zinc and trace elements are also needed. Zinc balances copper excess which may underlie depression, insomnia and aggressiveness. Calcium helps clear heavy metals, like lead, which cause hyperactivity, inability to concentrate and depression.

Certain amino acids are used in transmitting nerve impulses, but the best way to ensure balance is to take a full amino acid mix.

## Other Aids

Patterns of tension can be released using many of the physical therapies now available. Highly recommended are Chua Ka massage, Cranial Osteopathy, Feldenkrais.

Obviously the autonomic and central nervous system respond enormously to patterns of thought, feeling and perception. It is usually easier to start with physical healing here, but as the nervous system balances, you have to learn to recognise negative patterns, analyse and dispense with them.

You can start building more positive patterns by using the techniques of relaxation and visualisation. Breathing and exercise play a large part in the nerves because their energy supply is so critical. Many of the common drugs used, like barbiturates and tranquillisers, are very harmful in the long term, and should be avoided as far as possible.

References:
1. *Priest & Priest op. cit.*
2. *T. Yoshimoto et al. Flavonoids. Biochem. & Biophys. Res. Comm. 116(2). 1983.*
3. *Mrs. Grieve. op. cit.*
4. *C. Wright. The Wright Diet. Piatkus. 1986.*

# Herbal I        *Infection, Flu and Fever*

As well as for health promotion, useful in these conditions:

Abcess, bacterial invasion, cancer, fever, fungal infections, glandular fever, inflammation (e.g. laryngitis, bronchitis, meningitis and other - itis's) influenza, pneumonia, viral infections.
*(For any serious or lasting condition consult your practitioner.)*

| | | |
|---|---|---|
| **Comfrey** | root | *Symphytum officinale* |
| **Echinacea** | rootstock | *Echinacea angustifolia* |
| **Golden seal** | root | *Hydrastis canadensis* |
| **St. John's wort** | herb | *Hypericum perforatum* |

90mg as powder or per tablet except golden seal 70mg. 2-8 daily. Courses of no longer than 2 months. Golden seal reduces B vitamin synthesis in the colon, so supplement with B complex and have several months' break between courses.

## The Body

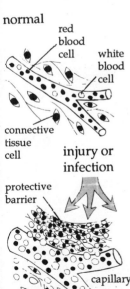

normal

red blood cell

white blood cell

connective tissue cell

injury or infection

protective barrier

capillary

size increases

We are normally insulated from infection by our impermeable skin, our active mucus membranes and the barrier of acid in the stomach. But many bacteria, viruses and fungi (e.g. Candida albicans) do find a home on and within the body, especially if there are wastes for them to feed on. If the invaders start multiplying and poisoning or killing the cells around them, the body goes into a protective inflammatory response. Body cells themselves may be damaged through toxicity or lack of protective nutrients and begin to reproduce themselves producing cancers or auto-immune imbalances. The body then reacts to these cells in a similar way.

First blood and lymph supplies to the area are increased, lymphocytes, the protective white cells, multiply, release antibodies and try to neutralise and engulf the invaders. 'Complement' in the blood itself enhances this response through chemical pathways. Connective tissue fibres mend and form a barrier around the area and may isolate it by making a cyst or abcess. If this is overwhelmed, the whole body goes into inflammatory response, increasing its temperature and mobilising all defences. The thymus gland and spleen hold reserves of lymphocytes which are released in times of need. The thymus releases a hormone thymosin

107

which stimulates antibody production and white T-cell activity. Many bacteria and viruses are less active at fever temperature, and can be cleared by a healthy protective system.

The inflammatory response is managed by the pituitary and adrenal glands, which are the same ones used in all stress situations. It is often when these are exhausted by other stresses, inadequate nutrition, addictions or drugs that the body fails to overcome infection. Excessive stress shrinks the thymus gland and reduces our capacity to resist "invaders".

Both wastes which attracted infection and the destructive poisons produced by viruses and bacteria must be cleared out. The first cleansing department is the lymph and its white cells, and infection is often contained in the lymph nodes, appendix and tonsils, as well as the larger vessels. But poisons eventually get to the blood and are treated by the liver. Then our organs of elimination take over and we need to help discharge toxicity through urine, faeces, sweat and mucus.

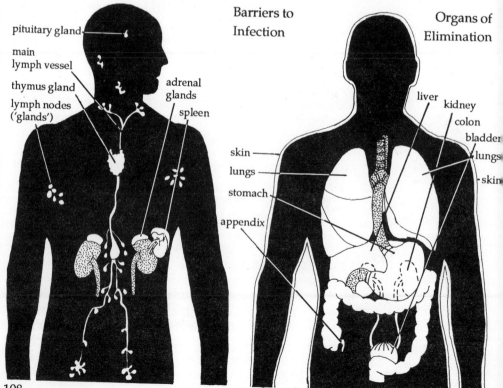

Barriers to Infection

Organs of Elimination

pituitary gland

main lymph vessel

thymus gland

lymph nodes ('glands')

adrenal glands

spleen

liver  kidney

colon

bladder

lungs

skin

skin

lungs

stomach

appendix

**The Combination**

Echinacea and golden seal are very powerful anti-bacterial, antiseptic agents. Comfrey, echinacea and golden seal detoxify and stimulate the lymphatic and blood circulation to increase flow and make white blood cells available.

All four heal wounds and local inflammation in skin and all mucus membranes and have been used externally as well as internally for this purpose. A spectrum of elimination enhancement is produced between the four, increasing the discharge of toxins through skin, lungs, colon and kidneys.

**The Herbs**
*Comfrey*

Comfrey root is mucilagenous and clears intestinal putrefaction and stimulates kidneys and lungs, increasing elimination. Its allantoin is known to stimulate the regeneration of cells, encouraging the repair of connective tissue. Comfrey is strengthening to liver, blood and lymph, helping to regenerate new tissue. It reduces excessive discharge, relieves pain, 'allays irritation' (1) and controls excessive temperature, thus balancing fever. Culpepper says that the leaves applied directly "heal running ulcers, gangrene, mortification" (2)

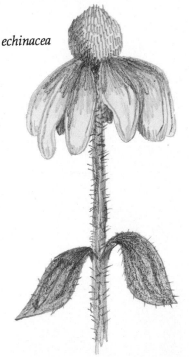

echinacea

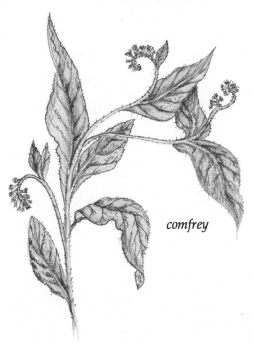

comfrey

*Echinacea*

Echinacea, one of the "succulent" healers is a supreme blood cleanser and direct anti-infection agent (3), to the extent of traditional use in stopping gangrene. It has been used successfully on a variety of serious infections and diseases, including typhoid, syphilis, cancer and diphtheria. It is said to encourage infective toxins to leave the body rather than being reabsorbed, and to have been effective in treating toxemia, septicemia and boils.

Current research (4) shows that echinacea stimulates the complement pathway through its major component, inulin, and enhances a variety of immune activities, like neutralisation of viruses and bacteria, migration of white cells to areas of infection, T-cell activation, interferon production, killer cell activity and antibody binding. It has specific antiviral activity against influenza and herpes, and also prevents the spread of such organisms in the body.

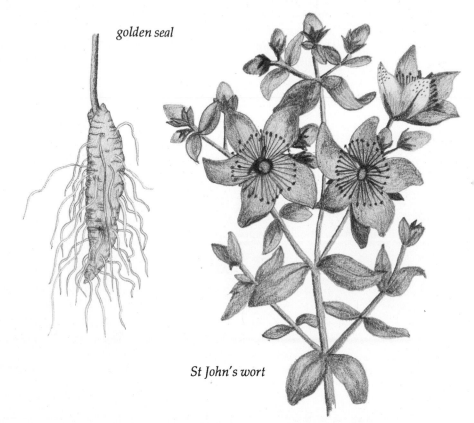

*golden seal*

*St John's wort*

*Golden Seal*

Golden seal, besides catalising other herbs, acts on mucus membranes, kidney, liver, lymph and glandular system as an antiseptic and soothing tonic. It is noted for dealing with skin diseases and "childhood infections" like chickenpox, flu and tonsilitis. Candida albicans, thrush and vaginal ailments and nasal or rectal irritation and infection have been treated with golden seal in dilute solution as well as by mouth. It has been shown to relieve diarrhoea even in severe gastro intestinal infections. It stimulates the immune system, particularly by activating the spleen, and by encouraging macrophages, the white cells that eat up bacteria, fungi, viruses and tumour cells (5).

*St.John's wort*

St.John's wort works largely on the nervous and glandular systems, calming and balancing the inflammation response. In fever it acts by reducing discharges and rebalancing metabolic rate. It also clears lungs, intestines and skin of toxins and improves circulation. St. John's wort has been used traditionally in tuberculosis and lung conditions, bladder infections, diarrhoea and intestinal worms. Its Greek name refers to its power over evil spirits!

**The Mixture**

The mixture contains heat and mineral strength in its watery antiseptic nature. It has an extraordinary sympathy with the skin and mucus membranes when one smells it.

**Nutrition**

"If you feed a cold then you'll have to starve a fever" is the way the old adage should be remembered. The worst thing to give the invading "germs" is a heavy meal.

For acute fevers, drink water, fruit and vegetable juices (not sweetened or preserved) and herb teas. Eat a little fruit or raw vegetables. Periodic fasts on fruit, vegetables or juices will help to clear general or long term infections.

Definitely avoid all heavy cooked food, preserved and processed food, sweets, biscuits, pastry, cakes, salty food and other "treats" as these will simply prolong the illness.

For cancer and other protective system breakdowns a clean and vital diet is essential and fresh carrot, beetroot and other vegetable and fruit juices should be taken frequently. Seek more information if you are dealing with such serious conditions.

As a rule sufficient good quality protein foods are essential to keep the immune system functioning well.

Vegetable protein is highest in seeds, grains and pulses. To get a good balance of amino acids, vary and mix these. For instance, combining rice and millet or rice and lentils makes a full complement of essential amino acids. Make sure that meat and dairy products are organically raised. The antibiotics, hormones, preservatives and bacteria in most animal products are prevalent and highly damaging to a weakened immune system.

Foods high in beneficial bacteria, such as natural yoghurts, sauerkraut and lactic fermented vegetables can help to restore a good bacterial population in the intestines and reduce the likelihood of infection coming from food or intestinal putrefaction.

## Supplements

The main anti-inflammatory vitamins which will also heal and detoxify are A (25-200,000iu, best as beta carotene) and C (2-20 grams). Zinc (50-100mg chelated) is the main mineral. Use the highest dosage only during short term acute infection for a few days. Selenium (50mcg) and organic germanium (5-50mg) are trace elements which have been found to boost the immune system. An amino acid complex will support the production and activity of white cells. As the bacterial balance of the intestines is also important as a basis for immune system health and recovery, you can clean and reestablish the intestinal flora using probiotic formulae - mixed beneficial bacteria.

Chlorella also has excellent immune-boosting, healing and detoxifying properties. Optimal dosage in these circumstances is 6 grams per day.

For glandular exhaustion an overall supplement programme should be boosted with B complex (75mg major B's), B5 (500-1500mg), C (3 grams), a multimineral, glandular extracts (thymus, adrenals and pituitary or a multiglandular extract) and ginseng or the Herbal Tonic combination.

For major protective system breakdowns this kind of programme is suitable in addition to the maintenance level of supplements; but you must take responsibility for your regime and work in consultation with your practitioner.

## Other Aids

Using antibiotics or fever supressors will drive the problem "underground" and you may have to deal with it later. Such drugs are only for the direst emergencies and even then, given in the correct doses, natural substances can be more effective than chemotherapy. For example the use of vitamin C is well documented (6).

Stay warm and relaxed during a fever. Mild infections may respond to heating the body, through exercise, sauna, blankets or steambath which will also stimulate sweating.

There is a great accumulation of evidence that the immune system can be strengthened using dietary factors, and serious diseases like cancer can be prevented and to a surprising degree treated using natural methods (7). Many of the natural therapies are applicable. The use of visualisation in cancer and serious protective system diseases has proved a great asset to the healing process, for example.

*References:*
1. *Priest & Priest. op. cit.*
2. *Mrs. Grieve. op. cit.*
3. *Priest & Priest. op. cit.*
4. *Dr. M. Murray. The 21st Century Herbal. Vita-Line. Contains several specific references to experiments.*
5. *M. Murray. Ibid.*
6. *E. Cheraskin, W.M. Ringsdorf Jr., E.L. Sisley. The Vitamin C Connection. Harper & Row. 1983.*
   *Irwin Stone. The Healing Factor. Grosset & Dunlap.*
7. *D. Dickenson. How to Fortify Your Immune System. Arlington Books. 1984.*

# Herbal K    *Weight Loss and Energy*

As well as for health promotion and as a trace mineral supplement, useful in these conditions:

Cold (feeling the...), depression, dull hair, skin and eyes, exhaustion, goitre, hypertension, lethargy, obesity, oedema, poisoning (heavy metals), sleep (excessive), thyroid (low), water retention, weight (excessive).
*(For any serious or lasting condition consult your practitioner)*

| | | |
|---|---|---|
| **Kelp** | herb (seaweed) | *e.g. Fucus* |
| **Alfalfa** | herb | *Medicago sativa* |
| **Dandelion** | root | *Taraxacum officinale* |

100mg of alfalfa and dandelion, 350mg kelp per tablet. 1-10 daily. As powder up to 800mg alfalfa, dandelion, 2.5 grams kelp daily.

**The Body**    Trace quantities of minerals are needed by the whole body to maintain full functioning. Processing, fertilisers and pollution ensure that our diet has become less and less adequate in the rarer minerals.

One particular mineral, iodine, is used to produce thyroid gland hormones, thyroxin and triiodothyroxin. These hormones control metabolic rate, or in other words our overall energy level, use of fat and sugars, feeling of warmth or cold, rate of healing and replacement of tissues. Low thyroid function is associated with low energy and lethargy, a tendency to put on weight, feel cold and have dull skin, hair and eyes. The thyroid gland of course is deeply associated with the other glands, and during the healing process its function may fluctuate over a period of months.

Every cell of the body has a "pump" which removes sodium and brings in potassium. The blood level of minerals is controlled by the kidneys in cooperation with the pituitary and adrenal glands. Excess sodium often taken as table salt, tends to increase water retention. This can lead to hypertension and blood pressure problems or to tissue storage of sodium, cellulite and swelling. It upsets the working of muscles and nerves and can irritate sensitive membranes like the nasal passages. The sodium pump, encouraged by more available

## Cell Diagram

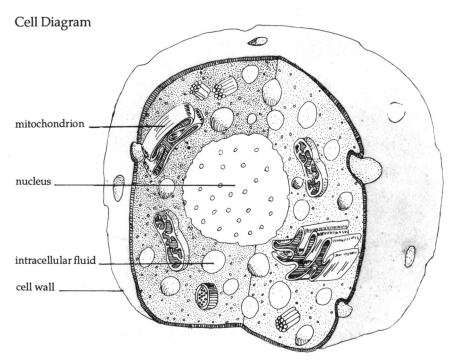

mitochondrion

nucleus

intracellular fluid

cell wall

energy and potassium will relieve each cell of irritating, water-pulling sodium and the excess will be discharged via the kidneys.

The energy centres of each cell, the mitochondria, contain all the enzymes needed for the gradual and careful "burning" of sugars and fats with oxygen to make energy for the sodium pump and all vital functions. Trace elements, vitamins and amino acids are essential to full mitochondrial function.

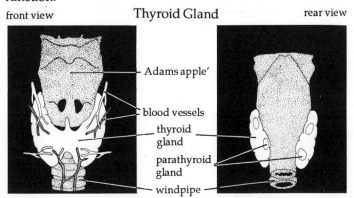

front view      Thyroid Gland      rear view

Adams apple'

blood vessels

thyroid gland

parathyroid gland

windpipe

Another aspect of importance to weight control and energy is our ability to digest foods fully. Failure to do this can lead to irritating particles within the body causing allergic reactions, swelling and water retention as well as exhaustion. So stimulation of the digestive enzymes as well as energy enzymes is important.

## The Combination

Together with kelp, alfalfa and dandelion provide a very wide and balanced range of trace minerals. They are an excellent source of natural vitamins and contain the essential amino acids. They gather their nutrients from the sea and the earth.

Kelp and dandelion cleanse the large intestine, liver and kidneys and help remove toxic chemicals. Digestion and assimilation is aided by all three. The sodium level is balanced by the potassium of dandelion and kelp.

## The Herbs
### *Kelp*

Kelp is the main constituent and provides the iodine strength to really boost metabolism, aiding thyroid function and promoting weight control, body heat and good hair, skin, nails and eyes. Areas of the world low in iodine have long been known for the incidence of severe thyroid problems, including cretinism, myxedema and goitre, but slight deficiencies are also common. From her studies of thyroid function, Dr. Barnes[1] estimates that the daily requirement of iodine is 0.21 mg a day. This compares with an average daily intake of 0.03 mg in an ordinary non-goitre region, and much less inside the goitre regions. Table salt may be iodised, but kelp gives us many other advantages, not least that sodium

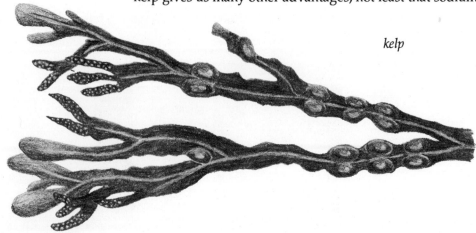

*kelp*

and chloride is naturally balanced with potassium and other necessary salts in kelp.

Kelp's alginate mucilage is cleansing and an aid to digestion and intestinal health. It filters the sea for minerals and provides us with a range which food from the land cannot match.

*Alfalfa*

Nutritionally a most complete plant food, alfalfa gives us enzymes to help digestion, complete proteins (including eight essential amino acids), high vitamin levels and good mineral content. It helps balance appetite, is a tonic and mild diuretic and an intestinal cleanser.

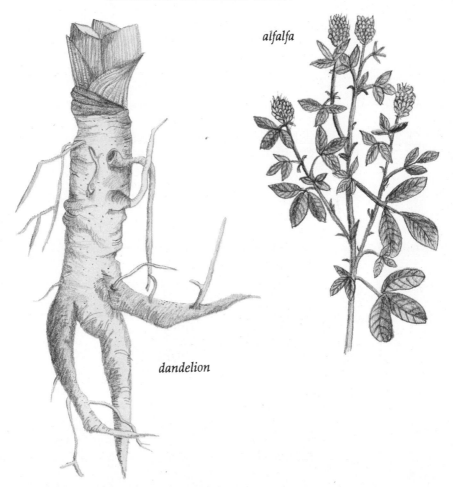

*alfalfa*

*dandelion*

*Dandelion*

Dandelion's deep root pulls nutrients from the soil and is an excellent source of organic potassium. This makes it good for weight control, particularly where water retention is involved. It is cleansing, diuretic and a blood builder. It strengthens and conditions the kidneys. In an experiment, animals were given fluid extract of dandelion root for a month. They lost as much as 30% of their original weight, much of it in the form of excess fluid (2).

**The Mixture**

The mixture is a strong green-brown with the strength of minerals and the smell of the sea and rich soil combined. It has the grounded power of water and earth.

**Nutrition**

A diet to speed metabolism is free of preservatives and toxic additives which undoubtedly slow and disrupt our biochemistry. High quality, natural sugars, fats/oils and proteins are the primary needs. This means avoiding sucrose sugar (especially refined), heavy sauces, heavy starchy food and overcooked food. Raw, fresh, fibrous, and whole food is energy promoting and weight reducing. Also avoid salt (which raises sugar levels and lowers liver function). The quality of calories is more important than quantity, and it is important to be healthy and lose weight rather than concentrating just on weight loss.

The Wright Diet gives further information on diet and supplements (3).

**Supplements**

In addition to the maintenance programme, the following supplements may be helpful:

The B vitamins are important for energy and conversion of fats. You might add to a B complex (75mg per major B vitamin) up to 500mg B6 if you have both fat and water retention, and especially if you are over-sensitive or tense.

Lecithin (2400mg) is a fat emulsifier, and is essential for fat transport and mobilising fat stores.

Digestive enzymes can be useful if extra weight is due to "bloating" or allergic reactions to incompletely digested food.

Besides the iodine in kelp, thyroid activity can also be balanced using a B complex particularly PABA (500mg) and raw glandular extracts. High protein diets should always be accompanied by extra A and E. High fibre diets, fasting on fruits, juices or other raw foods are methods that work well for natural weight loss.

## Other Aids

We would not recommend any artificial foods or treatments, which can present the body with real problems. Exercise and breathing are, of course, important. Getting the heart pumping and blood coursing and getting hot and sweaty once a day at least, really encourages weight loss and full metabolism. The exercise system Psychocalisthenics® is recommended.

Extra weight often goes with fears and anxieties, for instance about feeling loved. A full examination of the question "Why do I need extra weight?" and "Why do I need low energy?" can give great insight. Visualising that day by day you are returning to your correct weight and energy level will prepare the body properly for the herbs to do their work.

*References:*
1. B.O. Barnes, L. Galton. *Hypothyroidism: The Unsuspected Illness. Harper & Row.* 1976.
2. E. Racz-Kotilla, E. Racz, A. Solomon. *Planta Medica* 26:212-7. 1974.
3. C. Wright. *The Wright Diet. Piatkus.* 1986.

## Herbal M  *Mothers' Milk and Body Fluids*

As well as for health promotion, useful in these conditions:

Breasts (swelling, hardening), indigestion, insufficient milk, mammary cysts, carcinomas and infections, mastitis, mucus, obstruction of flow in blood, digestion, lymph and milk, skin and sweat gland problems.

*(For any serious or lasting condition consult your practitioner)*

**Fennel**    seeds  *Foeniculum vulgare*
**Fenugreek**  seeds  *Trigonella foenum graecum*

Up to 1 gram each of crushed seeds or 200mg of each per tablet. 2-6 daily.

**The Body**

Our bodies are made more of water than anything else, and we are entirely dependant on its management as a medium for transport and the chemical reactions of life.

Mothers' milk is an example of the importance of liquid as it passes from mother to child. We can focus on milk and the mammary glands, but equally we should look at the body fluids and liquid processes in both sexes.

Breast

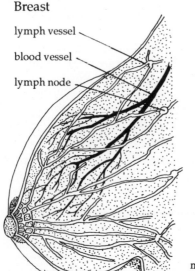
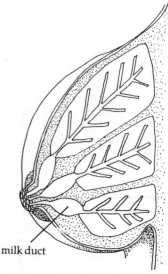

lymph vessel

blood vessel

lymph node

milk duct

Sweat Gland

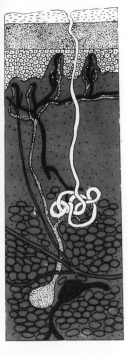

The mammary glands are modified sweat glands and develop their special secretory powers under the influence of hormones from the female pituitary gland. They change, as do sweat glands, with the menstrual cycle, and only start to produce milk when hormone balance changes following pregnancy and then birth. They are richly supplied with blood and lymph vessels which normally increase their activity when the rich foods are extracted for milk.

Problems with the lymph glands are symptomatic of the difficulty in the whole lymphatic system. The free flow of watery lymph and watery blood is an essential aspect of health.

Lactation draws our attention to other water secretions. The food of milk ultimately comes from the mother's digestive system which requires the right concentration of enzymes, acids and alkalis - all water based. If toxins are absorbed, they may travel the body in the form of watery mucus to build up in the lymph, skin, lungs or nose.

Lastly, the glands controlling lactation are deeply involved in the liquid balance of the body. The hormones they produce are water-borne secretions and hormone activity is very much to do with changing a target cell's relationship with its liquid environment.

## The Herbs
### Fennel

Fennel in its growth is designed for maximum flow of air and water with watery stems and warmth for its seeds. It is highly aromatic, and the anise-like oil stimulates digestion and lactation by encouraging secretion generally. It relaxes the smooth muscle of the mammary glands and calms abdominal pain by relaxing intestinal muscles. It helps balance pituitary functioning.

Fennel is useful in clearing lungs of mucus and intestines of gas, and according to Culpepper is "much help to open obstructions of liver, spleen and gall"[1]. It also keeps the lymph free of mucus and improves flow, helping to prevent cysts and cancerous growth.

Fennel helps to correct sodium/potassium balance, and hence water levels in the whole body.

### Fenugreek

Fenugreek's seeds are mucilagenous and are excellent for soothing digestion and dealing with mucus and water-borne toxins. It is effective in maintaining the delicate tubules of the mammary glands and clears lymph glands and lungs.

121

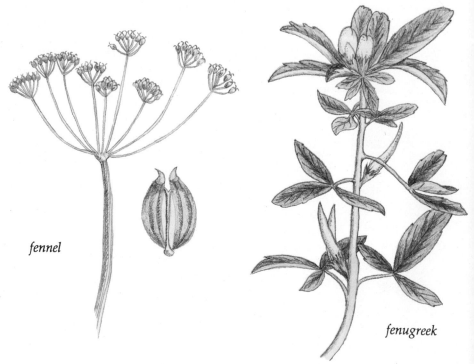

*fennel*

*fenugreek*

There is a long tradition of fenugreek restoring metabolism after illness, stress and pregnancy. It contains and promotes absorption of B vitamins, used in metabolism of nutrients and balancing the pituitary. There is some evidence from traditional use of more direct hormonal influence on lactation - for instance Sanecki says fenugreek "promotes lactation and encourages an alluring roundness to the bosom"[2]. It is much used in the Middle East for these properties.

## The Mixture

The mixture is a sweet aromatic mucilagenous light brown. It works mainly through the element of water, promoting clear flow. This is given fullness and good composition by the earthiness of fenugreek, and clarity and oxygenation by the airiness of fennel while the oils of both provide warmth.

## Nutrition

Liquids are taken into the body fluids quickly, and because of this we need to understand our own need for drinks. Obviously water, herb teas and juices are not a problem, but sugary, alcoholic and coloured, preserved and flavoured drinks are carried around the body and may diffuse into the tissues, including mammary glands, before they can be processed by the liver. Excessive coffee and tea drinking is directly linked to mastitis (breast cysts) (3).

Good quality foods will give the body what it needs to produce good quality secretions - this goes for nourishing milk, balanced hormones and odourless sweat!

So for alkalinity, minerals, enzymes and good sugars, use fresh raw vegetables and fruit. For protein eat fresh yoghurt, cheese, eggs, fish, mixed and sprouted grains, pulses and seeds, and avoid the preserved meats. For fats, eat in moderation dairy foods and butter, and cold pressed vegetable oils, not refined oils, animal fats or margarine. For starches, the long lasting energy source, we need whole grains and pulses, potatoes and bananas, and not white flour, cakes, bread and biscuits. Sweeten food with a little honey, molasses or fruit sugar, not white or brown sugar. Salt completely upsets the water balance and should not be used.

## Supplements

Water-carried vitamins and minerals can pass quickly into milk, and good all-round nutrition can be given to a child when mother uses supplements to maintenance level.

Cysts and other blockages respond to high A (25,000-100,000iu) best as beta carotene, and C (extra 1-5 grams), and mastitis to E (extra 400-3000iu providing blood pressure normal). If you are breast feeding keep to the lower end of this scale and consult your practitioner.

## Other Aids

Many mental and emotional blocks come to materialise in the breasts and lymphatics, particularly blocks in sexuality and early security, love and feeding patterns. Work with relaxation and visualisation of the tissues working smoothly and without blockage. Gentle massage and aromatherapy are excellent natural treatments. Exercise such as T'ai Chi, yoga or a relaxed use of the muscles will promote flow and balance of fluids in the body.

*References:*
1. *Mrs. Grieve. op. cit.*
2. *K.N. Sanecki. The Complete Book of Herbs. Macdonald & Jane's. 1975.*
3. *J.P. Minton. JAMA Medical News 24. 1221. 1979.*

# Herbal R    *Rheumatism and Arthritis*

As well as for health promotion, useful in these conditions.

Arthritis, bursitis, cramps, fibrositis, gout, joint pain, lumbago, muscle pain, rheumatoid arthritis, rheumatism. *(For any serious or lasting condition consult your practitioner.)*

| | | |
|---|---|---|
| **Alfalfa** | herb | *Medicago sativa* |
| **Burdock** | root | *Arctium lappa* |
| **Celery** | seed | *Apium graveolens* |
| **Comfrey** | root | *Symphytum officinale* |
| **Kelp** | herb | *Fucus vesiculosis* |
| **Sarsaparilla** | root | *Smilax officinale* |

65mg of each as powder or per tablet, 2-6 daily. Courses of no longer than 3 months.

**The Body**

Muscle tissue is made up of protein filaments which relax and contract in the presence of calcium and magnesium when this is initiated by a nervous impulse. Skeletal muscle is joined in bundles and covered by connective tissue which at its ends forms a strong connection or tendon to bone. Muscles span joints so that movement can be controlled. Joints are lined with cartilage and cushioned with clear lymph-like fluid. In normal relaxed movement the blood supplies sugars and oxygen which are the basis for energy production, plus the vitamins, minerals and raw materials for the numerous enzymes which control energy use in the muscles. It also helps to cleanse and renew cartilage and joint fluid, balancing the protein and mineral content.

However, during hard exercise, the blood contents are changed by the glands, and the needs of muscles and joints change too. Energy production may be "anaerobic" (without oxygen) producing lactic acid and an "oxygen debt" which must be repayed later. If acidic wastes are left in the body because of acidic diet or lack of vitamins needed to process them they may attract blood calcium and solidify in the muscles or joints.

Any stressful situation will provoke the pituitary gland to stimulate an adrenal stress reaction, raising blood sugar, fat and protein, diverting blood supply from skin and digestion to the muscles, raising blood pressure, and provoking release of calcium and other minerals into the blood.

Use of sugar, salt, tobacco, drugs, excess alcohol, or experiencing injury, fear, panic or great emotion, and crises of all kinds provoke stress reactions. If there is continual stress and any inadequacy in diet, wastes may be left in muscles, joints and the fine capillaries around them. Abnormal immune system reactions to this kind of imbalance can increase inflammation in the susceptible parts of the body.

Arthritic Joint                                    Healthy Joint

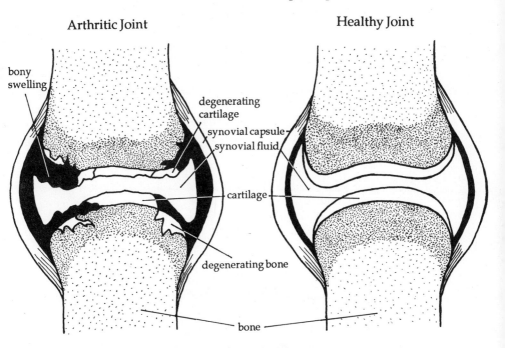

bony
swelling

degenerating
cartilage

synovial capsule
synovial fluid

cartilage

degenerating bone

bone

Wastes may include the residues of anaerobic respiration - lactic acid, uric acid. Cholesterol and fatty deposits may clog the capillaries, and calcium and other minerals may start to be laid down. In muscles this causes pain, stiffness and tension. In joints, there is pain, roughness, lack of movement and ultimately may be complete calcification. The drug cortisone has been used to try to rectify the long term effects of this arthritic process and reduce pain, but has proved highly dangerous to the health of patients. Adrenal cortisol (natural cortisone) is the body's own hormone treatment for pain and inflammation, and can be promoted by restoring the adrenals.

**The Combination**   Alfalfa, celery seed, kelp and sarsaparilla together provide a full range of minerals and trace elements, while aiding their assimilation from food. This encourages  glandular health and corrects mineral balance. Comfrey root and kelp are high in mucilage, which aids digestion and elimination in the intestines, raising the quality of foods in the blood and reducing wastes. Alfalfa, burdock and kelp  particularly, supply and aid the assimilation of vitamins needed for glands, energy production and tissue repair.

Celery, burdock and sarsaparilla stimulate the kidneys and tone the adrenals. They rebalance blood composition, and are known for their strength in blood cleansing.

**The Herbs**
*Alfalfa*

Alfalfa contains vitamins, such as vitamin C, which is required by the adrenal glands and in the correct formation of bone and connective tissue. It is also high in minerals, especially magnesium, used in balance with calcium in the body. It contains trace elements and eight essential amino acids. Alfalfa's digestive enzymes help to break down food

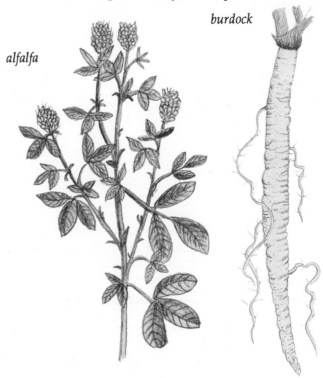

burdock

alfalfa

cleanly. It therefore helps to rebalance the glandular system and blood. It is well known in the USA as an arthritis aid and helps in the maintenance of joint and muscle tissue.

*Burdock*

Burbock root is one of the best blood purifiers, and "eliminates impurities from the blood very rapidly"[1]. It helps break down cholesterol and calcium deposits, and neutralise poisons. It is specific for reducing swelling in the joints and controlling inflammation and has a history of use for gout and rheumatism. It was used to prevent scurvy as it is a source of vitamin C.

*celery*

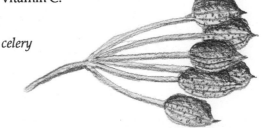

*Celery seed*

Celery seed is strongly diuretic and has a high mineral content. Its potassium would help to balance excess sodium for the health of the kidneys, adrenals and musculature. Its penetrating oils make it a powerful rheumatism remedy, and it has a history of reducing pain in neuralgia as well as rheumatism.

*Comfrey*

Comfrey root contains the powerful healer allantoin, which helps the repair of blood vessels and eases internal pains. It is used to help mend broken bones and has a great affinity for bone cell activity, normalising growth and use of minerals. Its other names - 'knitbone', and 'symphytum' (uniter) indicate the ancient tradition of use for bone problems. Comfrey's active constituent allantoin is known to stimulate healing of damaged tissues, and so would help with strained muscles, pulled tendons and pulled and damaged joints. Internal capillary haemorrhage into the synovial fluid of joints is often a feature of advanced arthritis, and Priest and Priest suggest that comfrey specifically helps capillary healing[2].

*Kelp*

Kelp is a promoter of glandular health, particularly helping the thyroid and adrenals. It increases supply of vitamins, minerals and trace elements drawn from the sea,

127

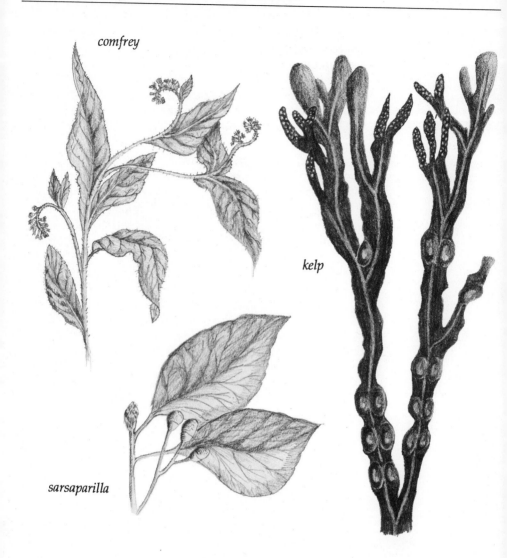

comfrey

kelp

sarsaparilla

which give the body the chance to build a full complement of enzymes necessary, to process rheumatic and arthritic deposits. Kelp has been used as a source of absorbable calcium to prevent rickets.

## Sarsaparilla

Sarsaparilla, well known blood cleanser and specific for rheumatism, also helps with glandular balance through its natural hormones. These help to buffer the stress reaction and allow the glands to heal. Sarsaparilla has a history of healing skin diseases and is particularly effective where there is both internal and external inflammation. It reduces the toxic load on the body by binding bacterial toxins from the colon (3).

## The Mixture

The mixture is sweet-sour and the aroma suffuses the body. It is brown-green and has the rebalancing strength of earth and mineral rich water. Sarsaparilla and celery carry the warming oils which penetrate dense tissue and bring relief.

## Nutrition

Salt (sodium) increases blood pressure, affects the composition of synovial fluid and alters mineral balance in blood and tissues. It encourages release of the inflammation-increasing hormones and elicits the stress reaction.

Sugar encourages blood sugar imbalance which elicits the stress reaction, strips the body of vitamins and upsets the mineral balance. Refined and heated oils and margarines make capillaries vulnerable to scarring and plaque formation.

People who suffer from bone, joint and muscle problems often have allergies and food sensitivities. If you are on a balanced diet and still having problems, you should take a look at this possibility. A simple self-administered sensitivity programme such as The Wright Diet (4) is recommended.

Diet for the arthritis/rheumatism area should include potassium-high green leafy vegetables and fruits, and slow releasing sugar sources such as whole grains, seeds and pulses, preferably sprouted, jacket potatoes and other whole starches. It should be highly alkaline (raw fresh fruit and vegetables, yoghurt and seeds are alkaline) to prevent calcium being withdrawn from bones into the blood. Fasting on non-citrus juices has proved very beneficial.

## Supplements

In addition to the maintenance supplement programme, anyone with problems in bones joints and muscles should consider using at least 4 grams of vitamin C a day (5). Acidic vitamin C can be replaced by a mineral ascorbate (e.g. magnesium ascorbate). Add to this extra B5 (pantothenate 500-1500mg) to help repair adrenal function and allow more cortisol to be produced. If your circulation is bad add C complex (bioflavonoids and rutin) and B3 (200mg) which will give you a skin flush and help clear capillaries. If your bones and teeth are at all weak add up to 6 dolomite with A & D tablets. Zinc is sometimes very useful for joint pain, particularly when there is copper excess.

Enzymes, particularly bromelain, can help bring down swellings and inflammation. The gamma linolenic acid in evening primrose oil (1000mg) or other GLA supplements helps to make prostaglandins which reduce inflammation.

To prevent post-menopausal osteoporosis supplementation with calcium, magnesium and boron (3mg) has proved effective.

**Other Aids**

There are many kinds of body work available which would address problems in this area. I would particularly recommend Chua Ka massage, Cranial Osteopathy and Feldenkrais. All the natural therapies have approaches and successes, and you need to find what works for you. Avoid using drug treatments, gold injections and cortisone treatment as far as possible. They tend to produce severe side effects and prevent natural healing.

Since emotions and mental blocks are stored in muscles, joints and their connective tissue, it is essential to release them during the course of healing. While massaging an affected area, or being massaged, allow memories and images to come up. Try to find the ones which still cause you pain, embarrassment or make you feel hot. Then use the technique in the introductory section, ending by visualising the affected place being suffused with soothing healing energy or light.

*References:*
1. *J. Kloss. op. cit.*
2. *Priest & Priest. op. cit.*
3. *M. Murray. The 21st Century Herbal.*
4. *C. Wright. The Wright Diet. Piatkus. 1986.*
5. *G.W. Campbell. A Doctor's Proven Home Cure for Arthritis. Parker. 1972.*

# Herbal S     *Sleep and Relaxation*

As well as for health-promotion useful in these conditions:

Fatigue, insomnia, jetlag, neuralgia, nightmares, overactivity, palpitations, stress, tension.
*(For any serious or lasting condition consult your practitioner.)*

| **Black cohosh** | root | *Cimicifuga racemosa* |
| **Catnip** | herb | *Napeta cataria* |
| **Hops** | flowers | *Humulus lupulus* |
| **Lady's slipper** | root | *Cypripedium pubescens* |
| **Scullcap** | herb | *Scutellaria galericulata* |
| **Valerian** | root | *Valeriana officinalis* |

Up to 300mg of each as powder or 50mg per tablet, 2-6 daily. Not to be used continuously at the high daily intake level.

**The Body**
The nightly cycle of sleep has two essential components. Firstly our muscles relax, breathing becomes regular, temperature falls and the eyes roll. Nervous activity, measured by EEG (Electro Encephalo Graph) goes by stages to the long regular rhythms of deep sleep. Then suddenly the eyes start to move rapidly, breathing and pulse rate become irregular and the muscles twitch and become flaccid. This

EEG

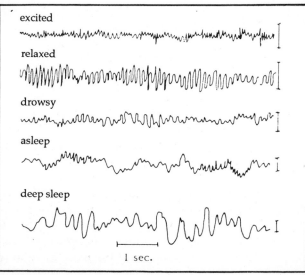

second part of the cycle happens when we dream, and it has been shown that this Rapid Eye Movement (REM) sleep is something we cannot do without.

Difficulty in sleeping starts with bodily discomfort - digestive and muscular pains, irritability in the sensory nerves or hormonal excitement. It has been shown that frequent waking is associated with adrenal hormone production which raises energy, pulse rate and all the natural functions.

The Brain

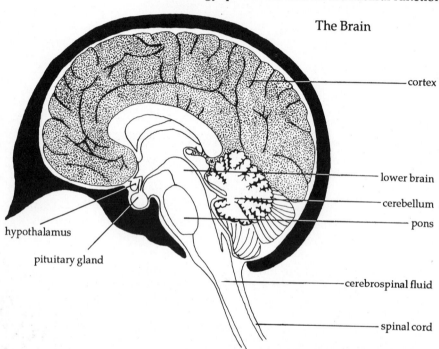

cortex

lower brain

cerebellum

pons

hypothalamus

pituitary gland

cerebrospinal fluid

spinal cord

But the other main area of control is in the lower brain, where breathing and autonomic functions are regulated. Here the amounts of neurotransmitters (nerve chemicals) like noradrenalin and serotonin are crucial. The chemistry of sleep is still largely unknown, however, and the reasons for the sedative effects of herbs are not well understood. But a number of herbal oils appear to act directly on the nervous system in the area of sedation, calming and reducing pain.

**The Combination**     Hops and catnip promote the digestive flow preventing disturbances from indigestion.

Black cohosh, hops, valerian and catnip soothe and encourage full blood circulation, preventing irregular pulse.

Scullcap, black cohosh, lady's slipper, valerian and catnip calm the musculature and are antispasmodic. All six herbs are nervine and gently sedative.

## The Herbs
### Black cohosh

Black cohosh reduces the pulse rate and has a calming effect on muscles and nerves. Herbalists have used it to treat delirium tremens, and have observed it to speed recovery from meningitis and it seems to relax the meningeal lining of the brain and restore cerebrospinal fluid [1]. It supplies natural hormones which help to balance the glands and prevent stimulating hormone production. It is a blood purifier, anti-toxic and anti-allergic preventing inflammation and disturbance.

### Catnip

Catnip is a remedy for colic and body pains in general. It prevents disturbance from fever and strengthens the glands against stress. It is calming and sedative, relaxing muscle tension and soothing the nerves. Jethro Kloss says of catnip, "If mothers would have this on hand... it would save them many sleepless nights"[2].

*black cohosh*

*catnip*

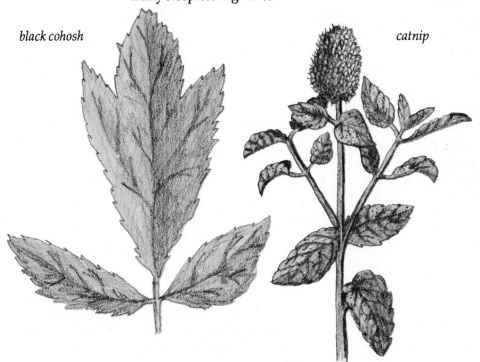

*Hops*

Hops are perhaps the best known of the combination for their promotion of the digestive enzyme flow, and their nervine and sedative properties. They will calm aches, fevers and nightmares. Hop-picking is such a pleasant occupation because of the soothing nature of hops. In an experiment rats were injected with a chemical extracted from hops which caused a 2 hour sleep 2 minutes later [3], with no side effects.

*lady's slipper*

*Lady's slipper*

Lady's slipper is valuable for its propensity for revitalising the nerves, while tranquillising and sedating. It is restorative, and has been used to calm hysteria and convulsions. It is known as American valerian and nerve root reflecting its history of use.

*Scullcap*

Scullcap is a tonic for the blood and a powerful nervine and antispasmodic. It soothes most nervous over-excitation and induces sleep without any unpleasant after-effects. It is well known for treating headaches, pains and irritations, like coughs, and was even used in epileptic fits.

*Valerian*

Valerian has been used to sedate the brain and nervous system in neuralgia and even St. Vitus Dance. It soothes pain and promotes sleep. Weak eyesight due to low energy in the optic nerve has been improved by valerian, pointing to its effect on dream (REM) sleep as well as deep sleep. It also calms palpitation and slows the heart. In an experiment on humans 400mg of valerian in water extract decreased sleep latency (waiting for sleep to come) and improved the quality of sleep especially amongst poor or irregular sleepers [4]. They were not especially sleepy in the morning and had unaffected dream recall.

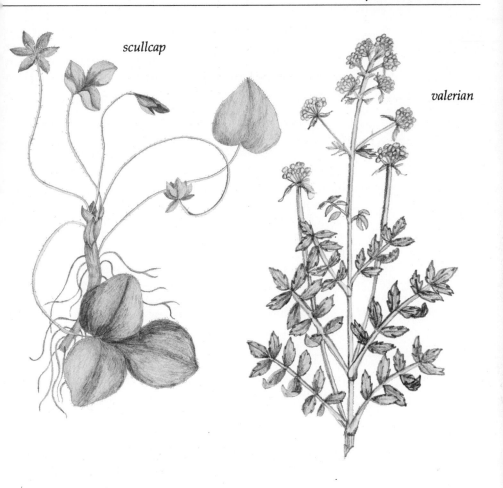

scullcap

valerian

**The Mixture**

The mixture's bitter-smooth smell fills the head with warmth and satisfaction and spreads slowly through the body. The colours are grey-green and it has the calming vibration of earth and water, which settle digestion and circulation.

**Nutrition**

Late eating and drinking is often disastrous for sleep. Digestive function slows during sleep, the bladder will slowly fill, and wind or the discomforts of indigestion can easily disturb.

Stimulating drinks such as cocoa, coffee, tea and alcohol (in its early stages) and sugary or salty foods will affect nerve, gland and muscle activity and prepare the body for action. The hormones of waking activity will effectively keep you from relaxation and sleep.

Food high in minerals, particularly calcium, are sleep-promoting. So the alkaline raw vegetables and fruits and milk, yoghurt and the lighter cheeses are good for the last meal of the day.

## Supplements

Calcium (4-8 tablets) as bonemeal, dolomite (with magnesium) or in chelated form is the place to start. It directly calms nerves and muscles. Zinc (50mg) is the second most important mineral as it balances the endless running-on of thoughts associated with copper excess. Magnesium (200mg) is needed to promote muscle relaxation.

As a rule vitamins are best taken during the active part of the day. If your sleep is colourless and you feel a lack of the refreshing dream cycle, though, B6 (100mg) will give you technicolour dreams. In fact, remembering dreams in colour is one way of testing whether you have enough B6.

B6 and B3 need to be present for the production of serotonin, the calming brain chemical. An amino acid L-tryptophan (300-1200mg) is the precursor of serotonin and is found to be an efficient sleep promoter.

## Other Aids

As we know, the mind and body are not truly separate, and if we cannot sleep because of one, the solution will usually be found in the other. For instance recurring thoughts running over the same lines often link with muscle tension. When there is some emotional problem the tension is usually found in the pattern of breathing. Learning to breath slowly, completely and comfortably through yoga or other time-honoured techniques can give you deep relaxation and mental release.

*References:*
1. *Priest & Priest. op. cit.*
2. *J. Kloss. op. cit.*
3. *R. Wolfhart et al. Planta Medica 48. 1983.*
4. *P. Leatherwood et al. Pharm., Biochem. & Behav. 17. 1982.*

Herbal T    *Tonic and Stimulant*

As well as for health promotion, useful in these conditions:

Lack of energy, muscle tone or vitality. Recovery from: accident, alcohol, antibiotic and other drug use, fatigue, infection, injury, innoculation, shock, stress, surgery, weakness.
*(For any serious or lasting condition consult your practitioner.)*

| | | |
|---|---|---|
| **Cayenne** | fruit | *Capsicum minimum* |
| **Dandelion** | root | *Taraxacum officinalis* |
| **Gentian** | root | *Gentiana lutea* |
| **Kelp** | herb | *Fucus vesiculosis* |
| **Nettle** | herb | *Urtica dioica* |

80mg each as powder or per tablet, 2-8 daily. Courses of no longer than 3 months.

**The Body**

Sometimes our body will go all out to fight off a disease or cope with a stress or accident. Sometimes we make it respond all-out by getting highly excited or competitive, or using alcohol or other drugs. Some of us have used a variety of means to extract the maximum from our bodies. Then when we have reached exhaustion, we really go downhill, often putting care for our bodies below other priorities.

In this state of depletion there is often lack of digestive enzymes and intestinal tone, leading to constipation, bad digestion and worse nutrition for the whole body.

Blood and lymphatic congestion and sluggish liver and kidneys are common. We become susceptible to minor infections of skin, urinary system and mucus membranes. Hair, skin and eyes become dull and nerves depressed. The glandular system, used excessively in stress situations, becomes exhausted and the balance between glands is lost.

The temptation when we're feeling low is to use the stimulants sugar, salt, caffeine, alcohol or drugs and go back into stimulating patterns like anxiety, overwork or verbal aggression.

The natural way of working is to encourage the cleaning of blockages, the production of enzymes and hormones, and the restoration of damaged or exhausted tissue. Certain herbs can aid this long term process while

137

providing an immediate boost to nerves and glands which makes us feel awake and alive.

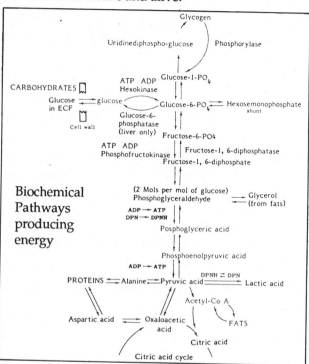

Biochemical Pathways producing energy

## The Combination

Gentian, dandelion, nettle and cayenne tone the digestive system and stimulate the production of enzymes, encouraging better nutrition for the tired body. Dandelion, kelp and cayenne cleanse, and rebuild the blood, and strengthen the heart and blood vessels, encouraging the use of protein in rebuilding tissue. Kelp and cayenne, aiding the use of vitamins and minerals, are restorers of the glands and nervous system.

Nettle and cayenne heal ulcerated or damaged tissue, and bring back the lustre of protein rebuilding in hair, skin and eyes.

Dandelion and nettle stimulate the kidneys.

Gentian and cayenne are antiseptic, preventing infection.

## The Herbs
*Cayenne*

Cayenne is a catalyst to other herbs and as a strong stimulant is useful for shock. It tones and heals the intestine and, with its vitamin C, iron and other mineral content, strengthens and cleanses the blood, and regulates heart rate. It wards off infection and stimulates all organs to full functioning, especially by improving blood supply to starved areas. "Capsicum is a pure stimulant, permanent in its action, and ultimately reaching every organ of the body"[1].

*Dandelion*

Dandelion is a mild laxative and stimulates digestion and appetite. Its high potassium content gives it diuretic properties and it cleans and strengthens both kidneys and liver. This reduces sodium (salt) storage which can slow down metabolism (salt is a preservative). Dandelion is a blood cleanser and provider of vitamins, minerals and trace elements.

*cayenne*

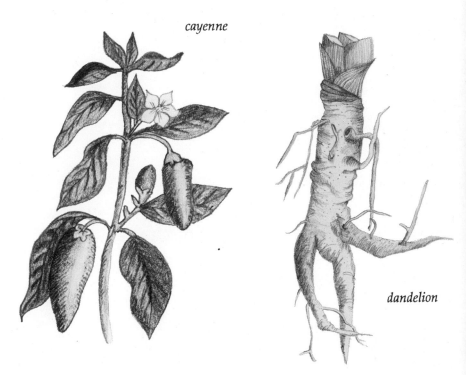

*dandelion*

*Gentian*

Gentian has long been known as a restorative in states of exhaustion. It acts on the delicate tissues of the digestive system and liver, protecting from infection and restoring normal activity. It has been used to aid recovery from jaundice and to eliminate intestinal parasites.

139

*Kelp*

Kelp's mucilage soothes digestion and encourages elimination of toxins. Its high mineral and trace element content encourages rebalancing of glands and nerves and restores the whole metabolism by aiding enzyme production. Low thyroid activity (hypothyroidism) is a common condition which lowers basal temperature and metabolism and may underlie problems from fatigue and low resistance to disease to glandular imbalance and depression (2). Kelp's iodine can help to rectify this condition.

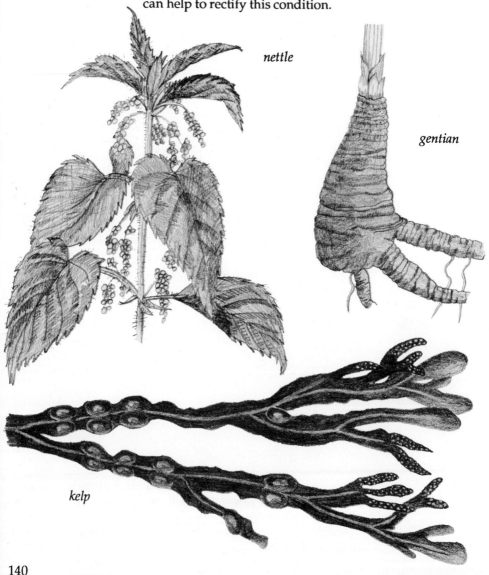

*nettle*

*gentian*

*kelp*

**Nettle**

Nettle, a traditional cleansing spring tonic, stimulates the kidneys and clears urinary ailments. Like cayenne it heals internal ulceration or bleeding. Because of its long roots it, too, contains many minerals needed by the body.

## The Mixture

The mixture of bright orange cayenne, bright green nettle, dark brown kelp and light brown dandelion and gentian, gives an indication of the power and wide spectrum of the combination. The smells are bitter and hot, and strongly awakening to the whole body. The earth element gives fiery stimulants their balance, and rhythmic water herbs their strength.

## Nutrition

Energy food is usually said to be sugar. But white or brown sugar is almost pure sucrose devoid of the other nutrients needed to make energy. In fact a diet high in sugar, salt, additives and preservatives is guaranteed to strip the body of essential nutrients and upset the production of energy and renewal of tissues.

Again we come back to fresh fruit and vegetables, and their juices. They are high in fruit sugar with a plentiful supply of necessary nutrients. Home-made soups too concentrate minerals, oils and proteins. The lighter proteins like pumpkin, sesame and sunflower seeds, yoghurt, low salt cheeses, fish and organic meat are recommended. Margarine, refined oils and animal fats will all deplete the body and cause problems, so cold pressed oils or virgin olive oil plus a little butter are more in tune.

To raise energy and avoid having to deal with waste we need the lighter starches - sprouted and boiled grain, whole potatoes. No mixtures like cakes and biscuits have been known to aid recovery and energy!

## Supplements

Exhaustion and debility often indicate a long term lack of vital vitamins and minerals, because of inadequate diet, stress or difficulties in absorption. Energy, rate of healing and recovery all depend on the essential nutrients to make the enzymes needed for full metabolism.

In this condition, food is simply not a sufficient source. Supplementation should include all the maintenance level plus extra vitamin C. A course of amino acids in combination can also help to restore energy and enzymes in the whole body.

**Other Aids**      Fresh air and gentle exercise; hot and cold water baths or showers; skin brushing; deep relaxation and meditation; good sleep and no stimulants; these are some of the effective aids to recovery. Cultivating optimism is quite hard in low energy states, but is a most dynamic aid. Imagine, "With each breath I feel more energy, more balance, more strength". Remember to give your body maximum attention to its needs, especially the need for time. Recovery can be very deep if not pushed.

*References:*
1. *J. Kloss. op. cit.*
2. *B.O. Barnes, L. Galton. Hypothyroidism: The Unsuspected Illness. Harper & Row. 1976.*

# Herbal XXX *Anti-Stress*

Useful in all stress-based conditions and as a tonic:
*(For any serious or lasting condition consult your practitioner.)*

**Siberian ginseng**   root   *Eleutheroccus*
**Korean ginseng**     root   *Panax ginseng*
**American ginseng**   root   *Panax quinquefolium*

Up to 400mg Korean, American, 1 gram Siberian daily, or 80mg Korean, American, 240mg Siberian ginseng per tablet, 2-5 daily. Courses of 3 months. Should not be used by women with heavy menstrual bleeding, and with caution if you feel over-energised.

**The Body**

In Part 1, stress was explained as a most important agent of imbalance. The whole body is affected by the reactions we have to stress, whether it originates in the way we see the world as worrying, or threatening, from the habitual use of sugar, salt, alcohol, drugs and other stimulants, from overwork or some internal imbalance or illness.

The brain and nervous system, especially the hypothalamus brain centre, monitors stress and the reaction is carried throughout the body by hormones from the pituitary gland and the adrenal glands. In a stress reaction blood levels of sugar, fats, including cholesterol, minerals and proteins are raised. This can cause problems. For instance, protein may be leached from the stomach causing ulcers, and the rise and fall in blood sugar produces strong mood and behavioural changes. Frequently we become addicted to a stressor because it temporarily raises blood sugar (hyperglycemia), making us feel super-human, only to have it withdrawn by an increasingly touchy pancreas (hypoglycemia), making us feel sub-human.

Adrenal hormones also manage inflammation and responses to infection. When adrenals are exhausted or out of balance, inflammations like arthritis and neuritis may set in, or the thymus gland's size may be so reduced as to undermine the effectiveness of protective white cells. In fact stress-induced failure of the adrenals underlies many chronic and degenerative diseases.

Really, the stress response is based on a very practical

143

way for the body to coordinate energy and the activity of all the organs and tissues to adapt to change. It should allow us to focus attention on a threat or a need for extra effort and stimulate the body to cope successfully. It should allow us to have a full and active life through to old age, and to be able to enjoy our food, our interaction with others, our sex life, physical strength and flexibility and all the normal strenuous activity of a full life.

**Energy Glands**

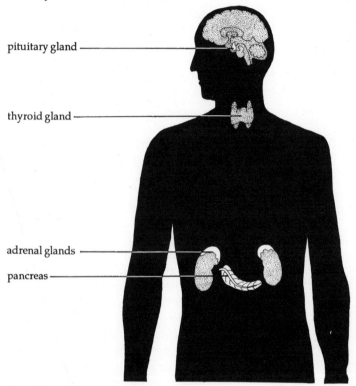

pituitary gland —

thyroid gland —

adrenal glands —

pancreas —

**The Combination**     Ginsengs are classed together because they all provide a tonic for glands, nerves, and muscles, increasing stress resistance and energy while allowing relaxation. They promote digestion. They certainly aid adaptation, and may promote rejuvenation.

**The Herbs**
*Siberian ginseng*

Though not a "true ginseng" this plant has proved exceptional in helping the body adapt to physical stress. Professor Breckman described a number of exciting Russian experiments [1]. A test of athletes over a ten mile race showed

144

that those who had taken eleutherococcus ran on average five minutes faster than those on a placebo. Flu and colds after stress were reduced in a survey of 1000 workers taking daily ginseng and various aspects of resistance to illness were improved. With later experiments they found that the glycosides of eleutherococcus abolished the alarm (adrenaline) reaction in animals who were sent swimming. They also went on swimming longer, but this was not at the expense of an adrenal stress reaction, and in some animals the level of cortisol in the blood actually fell. Other effects include improved dark-adaptation of the eye, visual acuity, colour perception and hearing. So-called 'adaptogens', similar to those in the other ginsengs, give it a wide range of beneficial effects on glands and nerves, particularly toning the pituitary and adrenal glands. Chinese scientists report that it reduces general fatigue and weakness in 90% of patients [2].

*Korean ginseng*

The best quality white Panax root is prized by Eastern connoisseurs. It has been found to have strong effects on body processes which are mediated by hormones while actually strengthening and balancing the glandular system. It helped diabetic mice to make more insulin and lower their blood sugar level without raising adrenalin or stressing the pancreas [3]. It appears to reduce inflammations generally and

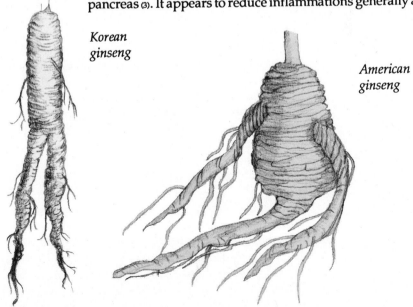

*Korean ginseng*

*American ginseng*

145

amplify the effects of the cortisol family of adrenal hormones without side effects [4], and this is achieved without raising blood sugar [5].

Panax has been discovered to enhance immunity, for instance it protects mice from a virus which is normally lethal [6] and from normally damaging X-ray radiation [7].

Research shows that Panax ginseng stimulates the body's ability to carry through energy production via the anaerobic route, through lactic acid [8]. Older people are thought to lose the capacity to use all their food for energy in this way, and this might explain some of the rejuvenating effects observed.

It helps normalise menstruation and may aid childbirth. Korean ginseng has made people feel so good that they think of it as an aphrodisiac. The adrenals also produce sex hormones, which may explain this. It is helpful in coughs and chest ailments as well as stomach and digestive difficulties.

*American ginseng*      Current research emphasises its calming, tranquillising, almost sedative effects [9], but it has been prized on the Eastern market as an equal to Korean. It was used by American Indians to prevent nausea and vomiting. It provides a good balance to Siberian ginseng by toning down the stimulating effects.

All ginsengs lower serum cholesterol and fats [10], and American has been found to increase the proportion of the safe and necessary HDL component relative to the dangerous LDL cholesterol implicated in circulatory diseases [11].

**The Mixture**      The mixture is a rich light brown with the harder brown of Siberian modified by the creamier colours of Korean and American. Warmth and earthiness. The roots absorb so much from the soil that it is said they can never be grown in the same soil twice. The real ginsengs take up a certain quality of light which can make them glow.

**Nutrition**      Eating for stress is a matter of supporting the body's normal energetic activity while breaking the cycles of over-stimulation and exhaustion.

Sugar addiction should be stabilised by substituting honey, molasses and fruit sugar for all white, brown and added sucrose sugar, and using slow-releasing starches like potato, sprouted pulses and whole grains and bananas or plantains. Salt addiction must be halted, and vegetable concentrates or naturally salty vegetables like celery are good substitutes.Additive and preservative-rich food should be exchanged for fresh raw fruit and vegetables, fish, cheese, eggs, rice and lentils and fresh meat. Animal fats and processed oils, including margarine can be damaging and ageing, especially to the circulatory system, and should be replaced by cold-pressed sunflower or virgin olive oil on salads, and less fried food. Tea, coffee and alcohol, as well as sugary drinks, can enter the stress reaction and herbal teas, juice, water and dandelion coffee are good substitutes.

## Supplements

Specific for the stress reaction are B5 (500-1500mg) vitamin C (2-5 grams) and lecithin (2-4 grams). They should be taken with the maintenance programme.

Raw glandulars, particularly adrenal, pituitary or mixed glandular extracts are very fortifying, and mixed amino acids can also provide a considerable boost to the whole body during stress.

## Other Aids

Understanding that challenges are meant to be met with a healthy adaptation response will help you stop over-responding when it's not appropriate. Specialised stress reduction techniques may be useful, but the basis for dealing with stress in the moment is breathing, relaxation and centring. It is essential to find ways of dealing with the emotional background to stress, through therapy for instance.

*References:*
1. *Prof. Breckman. Inst. Marine Biology. USSR. Lecture Oct 1979.*
2. *M. Murray. The 21st Century Herbal. Vita Line.*
3. *M. Kimura et al. J. Pharm. Dyn. 4 1981.*
4. *S. Chong et al. Int. Arch. Allergy & App. Immunology. 73. 1984.*
5. *S. Hiai et al. Chem. Pharm. Bull. 31. 1983.*
6. *V. Singh et al. Planta Medica 47. 1983.*
7. *A. Takeda. J. Radi. Res. 23. 1982.*
8. *G. Shia et al. Gerontology 28. 1982.*
9. *S. Fulder. The Root of Being. Hutchinson. 1980.*
10. *A. Qureshi et al. Atherosclerosis 48. 1983.*
11. *Shultz et al. Fed. Proc. 39. 1980.*

# Part Four

## Appendices

# Nutritional Supplements

**Vitamin A**

Forms - beta carotene, *plant source:* Red and yellow vegetables.
Retinol (-yl acetate) *animal source:* Animal and fish liver.
Retinyl palmitate, non-animal form.
Retinol has been found to be toxic at high levels of dosage, but 20,000iu daily for life is said to be safe by the Government recognised Dunn Nutritional Laboratory. Levels above 50,000iu should be used only for a matter of days or should be well supervised. Beta carotene is non-toxic as it is converted to retinol within the body as needed.

**B Complex**

*Sources:* yeast, rice bran and other grains.

Maintenance levels (M) healing levels up to (H).

|  | M | H |
|---|---|---|
| B1 Thiamin | 10-75mg | 500mg |
| B2 Riboflavin | 5-75mg | 500mg |
| B3 Nicotinic Acid *(Niacin)* | 20-100mg | 5,000mg |
| B5 Pantothenic Acid | 20-100mg | 1,500mg |
| B6 Pyridoxin | 10-75mg | 600mg |
| B12 Cyanocobalamin | 5-50mcg | 5,000mcg |
| Folic Acid | 20-100mcg | 2,500mcg |
| Choline | 5-50mg | 1,500mg |
| Inositol | 5-50mg | 1,500mg |
| Lecithin *(high in choline and inositol)* | 50-1000mg | 15gm |
| Biotin | 5-50mcg | 300mcg |
| PABA | 10-100mg | 1000mg |

Always use a B complex back-up if using any of the single B's beyond maintenance level. Use sustained release for all-day coverage.

**C Complex**

*Sources*: rosehips, acerola cherries, peppers, oranges.

|  |  | M | H |
|---|---|---|---|
| Vitamin C ascorbic acid |  | 250mg-5grams | 20grams |
| Bioflavonoids |  |  |  |
| Hesperidin | Dietary | 2gm 10mg | 5grams |
| Rutin |  |  |  |

Quercetin is a bioflavonoid which reduces allergic reactions in some people quite dramatically. 250mg - 1000mg.

**Vitamin D**

Obtained from sunlight on the skin, dairy products, animals and fish,especially liver e.g. cod liver oil.

When calcium absorption is low and there is a lack of sunlight and low dietary sources of D, supplemental amounts may be useful (usually in combination with vitamin A).Up to 1000iu daily (H).

**Vitamin E**

*Sources:* grains, wheatgerm, seeds, nuts, cold pressed oils. Only natural d-alpha tocopherol (or tocopheryl acetate) is fully active. Avoid mixed tocopherols and synthetic E.

**Caution:** Heart and circulation patients should be cautious as high levels of E given without a slow build up can overstimulate heart and raise blood pressure. Start below 200iu daily and increase over 1-2 months to 400iu, doubling again after 1-2 months. Maintenance levels 200iu, healing levels 400-2000iu.

**E.F.A's - Essential Fatty Acids**

*Sources:* cold pressed oils, seeds, whole grains, nuts. Best taken as food. Vitamin E helps to conserve the essential fatty acids.

**G.L.A. - Gamma Linolenic Acid**

Gamma linolenic acid may be difficult for some people to make internally. It boosts the prostaglandins which control and reduce inflammation, pain and stress. *Sources:* evening primrose oil, black currant seed oil, borage seed oil.

**Calcium**

*Sources:* seeds, vegetables, dairy foods.
Supplemental Amounts: Maintenance 300-800 mg.
For healing up to 3000mg
as dolomite, bonemeal or amino acid chelated mineral, orotate or ascorbate. Requires vitamin D and A for absorption and use.

**Magnesium**

*Sources:* green vegetables, milk, nuts, whole grains.
Supplemental amounts: Maintenance 100-400mg.
For healing up to 1500mg
as dolomite, ascorbate, amino acid chelate, orotate.

**Potassium**

*Sources:* vegetables, fruit, seaweed.
Supplemental amounts:   Maintenance up to 50mg.
For healing up to 800mg
as Herbal K, amino acid chelate, orotate, ascorbate.

**Zinc**

*Sources:* eggs, cheese,oysters, whole grains (preferably sprouted).
Supplemental amounts:  Maintenance up to 10mg.
For healing up to 200mg
as amino acid chelate, orotate, ascorbate.

**Iron**

*Sources:* green vegetables, fruit, blood.
Supplemental amounts:  Maintenance up to 10mg.
For healing up to 80mg
as amino acid chelate, orotate (do not use inorganic iron).

**Other Minerals**

| | *source* | *upper healing level* | *supplement* |
|---|---|---|---|
| **Manganese** | buckwheat, grains | 100mg | amino acid chelate, ascorbate, orotate. |
| **Copper** | apricots, liver | 6mg | ditto |
| **Iodine** | kelp, seaweed | 2mg | kelp or ditto |
| **Chromium** | yeast, molasses | 800mcg | yeast or ditto |
| **Selenium** | garlic, onions | 200mcg | ditto |
| **Boron** | kelp, alfalfa, apples | 3mg | calcium Boro-gluconate, amino acid chelate |
| **Germanium** | garlic, onions | 250mg | citrate-lactate |
| **Trace Minerals** | seaweed | trace | kelp or amino acid chelate |

**Other Useful Supplements**

**Raw glandular extracts.** Low temperature extracts of carefully selected animal glands.
**RNA 500mg DNA 50mg** from yeast
**L-glutamine** amino acid
**Other amino acids** and complexes
**Digestive enzymes**
**Acidophilus**
**Probiotic and symbiotic bacteria** - beneficial intestinal flora
**Chlorella**
**Green barley**

# The Author

Brian Wright completed a Psychology degree at Sussex University in 1971 and left the academic world for the raw experience of counselling young drug addicts. This led to extensive investigation of the human potential movement and training at the Arica Institute, founded by Oscar Ichazo.

Since 1977 he has studied nutrition and many aspects of natural health enhancement with an emphasis on developing self knowledge and intuition.

Other books by the author:

**Cleansing the Colon.** *Green Press.*

with Celia Wright:

**The Nutrition Handbook.** *Green Press.*
**The Nutrition Programmes Handbook.** *Green Press.*

# Bibliography

**Herbs**

Hudson, Paul. 1977. *Mastering Herbalism*. Abacus, London.
Macleod, Dawn. 1968. *A Book of Herbs*. Duckworth, London.
Pelikan, Wilhelm. *Part 1. Healing Plants*. Rudolf Steiner Press,
Reprinted from The British Homoeopathic Journal.
   Facinating way of seeing the energy of plants in relation to people.
Grieve, M. 1977. *A Modern Herbal*. Penguin, England.
   *The* herbal encyclopaedia.
Garland, Sarah.1979. *The Herb and Spice Book*. . Frances Lincoln.
Fulder, Stephen. 1980. *The Root of Being. Ginseng*. Hutchinson. The
most comprehensive and well written book on ginseng available.
Sanecki, Kay N. 1975. *The Complete Book of Herbs*. Macdonald and
Jane's.
Royal, Penny C. 1978. *Herbally Yours*. Biworld, Utah, USA.
Kloss, Jethro. 1974. *Back to Eden*. Lifeline Books, California.
   A classic of American folk-medicine
Lust, John. 1978. *The Herb Book*. Bantam Books, New York.
Lewis, Walter H. & Memory E. 1977. *Medical Botany*. Plants Affecting
Man's Health. Wiley- Interscience, New York.
Gordon, Lesley, 1980. *A Country Herbal*. Webb & Bower, England.
Priest, A.W. and L.R. 1982. *Herbal Medication*. L.N.Fowler and Co.
Murray Dr. M. *The 21st Century Herbal*. Vita Line. U.S.A.
   A modern practical guide to herbal medicine.

**The Body**

Jolly, Richard T. 1980. *The New Atlas of the Human Body*. Corgi,
London. Beautifully illustrated.
Bevan, James 1978. *Anatomy and Physiology*. Mitchell Beazley.
Kessel, Richard G & Kardon, Randy H. 1979. Freeman, San Francisco.
McNaught & Callander. 1975. *Illustrated Physiology* Churchill
Livingstone. Understandable textbook.
Nilsson, Lennart. 1974. *Behold Man*. Harrap, London.
   Pictures to give a sense of the wonder of the Human Body.
Darwin, Charles, *The Origin of Species*, Penguin, Everyman.

**General**

Rolf, Ida P. Rolfing *The Integration of Human Structure*, Harper and
Row. An insight into the workings of human bodies by an innovator
and great healer.
Selye, Hans, 1978. *The Stress of Life*. McGraw Hill. USA.
   The father of the unified concept of stress gives a clear presenta-
tion of the mechanisms and some solutions.
Wright, Brian & Celia, 1979. *The Nutrition Handbook*. Green Press,
England. A simple presentation of basic principles of nutrition,
healing, fasting, supplements and the origin of a new perception of

health.

Wright, Celia. 1986. *The Wright Diet*. Piatkus.

A practical and informative presentation of diet and nutrition for individuals.

Rawson, Philip and Legeza, Laszlo, *Tao*. Thames & Hudson 1973.

A lavishly illustrated book on the basics of Taoist thought and practice.

Ichazo, Oscar. *Between Metaphysics and Protoanalysis*. Arica Institute Press. 1982.

This book provides some of the philosophical background to Oscar's great achievements in providing spiritual impulse and a scientific method through Arica. His analysis will, I am sure, be recognised as the basis for unified thought in science, humanities and all human activity. See also

*Interviews with Oscar Ichazo*. Arica Inst Press. 1982.

Current information about the Arica School and its trainings from Brian Wright, author.

Mann, Felix. *Acupuncture*. Pan Books. London 1971.

A basic introduction to Acupuncture theory and practice.

Pfeiffer, Carl C. *Mental and Elemental Nutrients*. Keats.1975.

A great textbook on the use of minerals and some vitamins, especially for mental/emotional health. Excellent source material.

J.I. Rodale and Staff. *The Complete Book of Minerals*. Rodale. 1976. Readable tome with much useful information.

Gerras Charles. *The Complete Book of Vitamins*. Rodale. 1977.

Companion volume to the Book of Minerals.

Zukav Gary. *The Dancing Wu Li Masters*. Bantam 1979.

One of the best of the recent books on the interface between ˙ysics and metaphysics.

˙sley David V. *Subtle Body*. Thames and Hudson. 1977.

A well illustrated book about etheric and other higher physical energies. His other books on Radionics and other aspects of healing are also recommended.

Wright, Brian. *Cleansing the Colon*. Green Press, England 1987.

**Other Recommended Authors**

Airola Paavo. *Nutrition and Self-help healing*.
Stone Irvin. *Vitamin C, The Healing Factor*.
Passwater Richard. *Diet and Healing*.
Hoffer Abram. *Vitamin Therapy*.
Bland Jeffrey. *Current Nutrition Research*.

# Index